# Ramy Gafni's
# Beauty Therapy

# Ramy Gafni's Beauty Therapy

The ultimate guide to looking and feeling great while living with cancer

## Ramy Gafni

M. Evans and Company, Inc
New York

## DISCLAIMER

This publication is designed to provide accurate and authoritative information in regard to the subject matter covered. It is sold with the understanding that the publisher is not engaged in rendering professional services. If medical, psychological, or any other expert assistance is required, the services of a competent professional person should be sought.

The information, ideas, procedures, and suggestions contained in this book are not intended to replace the services of a trained healthcare professional or to serve as a replacement for professional medical advice and care or as a substitute for any treatment prescribed by your physician. Matters regarding an individual's health often require medical supervision. A physician or health-care professional should be consulted regarding the use of any of the ideas, procedures, suggestions, or therapies in this book. Any application of the information set forth in this book is at the reader's discretion. The author and publisher hereby specifically disclaim any and all liability arising directly or indirectly from the use or application of any of the products, ideas, procedures, therapies, or suggestions contained in this book and any errors, omissions, and inaccuracies in the information contained herein.

Trade names are included for identification purposes only, and are not intended to endorse the product.

M. Evans and Company, Inc.
216 East 49th Street
New York, NY 10017

Library of Congress Cataloging-in-Publication Data
Gafni, Ramy.
[Beauty therapy]
 Ramy Gafni's beauty therapy : the ultimate guide to looking and feeling great while living with cancer / Ramy Gafni.
 p. cm.
 ISBN 1-59077-066-8
 1. Cancer in women--Palliative treatment. 2. Beauty, Personal. I. Title.
RC281.W65G34 2005
616.99'406--dc22

                    2005006807

*Typeset and Designed by Chrissy Kwasnik*

Printed in United States of America

9  8  7  6  5  4  3  2  1  0

## DEDICATION

To my parents, Sam and Rachel Shmuelof; my sister, Dina;
Eli and Maya. To Michelle Frohman Roth and Michael Snyder,
my dearest friends who have been there for me through it all,
and to all the people brave enough to face the world when
undergoing adversity as well as the guardian angels who help
them and make the world a better place.

# CONTENTS

# FOUR Face Time. Making Up Your Face

# FIVE Eyebrows and Eyelashes

# SIX Covering Up Chemotherapy and Radiation Side Effects

# SEVEN Beauty Therapy Rituals

# ACKNOWLEDGMENTS

I have been fortunate to encounter many people both professionally and personally who have been like guardian angels to me. This book would not have been possible without the collaboration of all the wonderful people at M. Evans and Molly Ward. I would especially like to thank Linda Konner, who was able to do what the giants in her field were not able to accomplish, and PJ Dempsey, who sees the forest, not just the trees. It has been a long and winding road from the moment over 6 years ago when I had the idea for this project to its ultimate completion. Thanks to my parents, Sam and Rachel. Dad, who taught me to dream big, and Mom, who taught me to work hard to achieve those dreams. Thanks also to Dina for making sure I do everything right.

A special nod to some guardian angels I met along the way who helped nudge this book along: Mel Berger, Neeti Madan, and Jack Scovil.

Thank you also to all the models in this book who are selfless enough and brave enough to show the world that a beautiful face is still beautiful, even when faced with adversity.

Sources:

Dr. Phoebe E. Rabbin, dermatologist in practice in New York City. She is a fellow of the American Academy of Dermatology and a diplomate of the American Board of Dermatology.

Emily Spivak, founder and executive director, Shop Well with You, a national not-for-profit organization that helps women with a history of cancer improve their body image and quality of life by using clothing as a means toward wellness. (www.shopwellwithyou.org).

Credits: Models photographed by Sioux Nesi. Photos have not been retouched.

Assistants to Sioux Nesi: Sebastian Kriete and Andrew Tingle

Styled by Stella Brandt

Makeup by Ramy Gafni

Hair by Cesar Ramirez for Dop Dop Salon

Hats generously loaned by Barbara Feinman (www.feinmanhats.com)

Illustrations by Albert Crudo (www.AlbertCrudo.com)

# FOREWORD

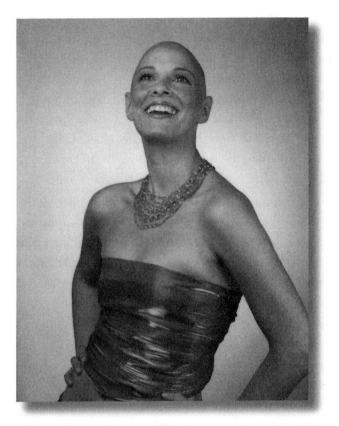

I knew even before reading the first chapter that this book would be special and valuable because of its author's enormous empathy and compassion. Ramy is a makeup artist, yes; but first, he is an extraordinary human being—kind, sensitive, intelligent, conscientious, easygoing, and downright adorable. I don't mean to make him sound like a boy scout—no, he is certainly not that—but who better to write this book? Given the subject matter, coping with the challenges to appearance and self-esteem that cancer treatment can bring, it seems most important and relevant that Ramy knows what he is writing about and that he cares about people, especially cancer sufferers and survivors, because he is a survivor himself; he is also a fine artist with a knack for simplifying the way-too-complex world of color cosmetics in order to help us look our best.

He first did that for me (a makeover) in 1996 when I was beauty editor at *Self* magazine. I was on a routine market appointment at a New York salon and was ushered to the counter where Ramy presided. We hit it off right away. I liked his philosophy and style; he was refreshingly sensible and informal. In a business that can be superficial and that often takes itself too seriously, he was direct and amazingly quite tender (a brave thing to be in this city). Hardly a tough New Yorker. And just the guy to show me how to do my makeup. I learned a lot and made a lifelong friend during that first visit.

After his treatment for non-Hodgkin's lymphoma, it came as no surprise to me that Ramy began doing makeup applications for other cancer patients gratis. I admit, I kept hoping he'd have very few takers. But unfortunately, cancer strikes over a million Americans each year, and we are all touched by the disease, knowing people who've fought it, lived through it, died from it.

Ramy's book is a loving gesture, a way of giving back because he knows what it is like to experience cancer, as well as to be lucky enough to survive it. He understands the healing power of beauty to help cancer patients look and feel their absolute best. No dictates, no expectations of perfection, no pressure to pretend you're not sick. Just support, artistry for the real world, and grace. For men and women struggling with cancer and its interruption in their lives, here is a book to give them strength—and more than a few great tips.

—JANET CARLSON FREED

BEAUTY AND HEALTH DIRECTOR, *Town & Country* MAGAZINE

# INTRODUCTION

What is beauty therapy? The dictionary defines these two words as follows: Beauty as a pleasing quality associated with harmony of form or color; therapy as (1) the treatment of an illness or disability; (2) a healing power or quality.

At first glance, it seems unlikely that anyone would combine these two words, but for me it makes perfect sense because beauty therapy is not about beauty as physical perfection. It is about creating beauty to help you look and feel your absolute best. When your world is turned upside down by cancer, looking like a supermodel doesn't even make your list of concerns; however, applying makeup or pampering yourself with a beauty ritual can work wonders for your self-image, your self-esteem, and your overall health and well-being. Whatever you do, even minimal things such as wearing concealer to hide the dark circles associated with sleeplessness from chemotherapy or radiation, or taking an aromatherapy bath to relax your mind and spirit, can help perk you up and be therapeutic during this extremely trying time. Any beauty ritual—getting a facial or exercising, or even shopping or listening to music—can make you feel renewed, stronger, and more positive. Believe me, a beautiful model diagnosed with cancer faces the same issues and fears as everyone else, and the pressure to look fit, healthy, and vibrant is greatly magnified when you earn your living based on your physical appearance.

When people are being treated for cancer, their self-image is often shattered. Cancer treatments are both a blessing and a curse. The very treatment that can save your life can also change your physical appearance, sometimes in traumatic ways. Suddenly, not only are you fighting for your life, but you are doing it while a stranger is staring back at you from the mirror. Your hair is gone, your nails are brittle—everything changes, even your eyebrows and eyelashes. All these changes attack your self-image and go to the very core of your physical and sexual identity.

This book will help you to literally put on a new face and get through this ordeal. How can a beauty book do this? Well, when we look good, we feel good. Putting forward a good face helps us take on the world in a positive way.

I know that firsthand. I've been there. I am a makeup artist who was diagnosed with stage I B-cell sclerosing mediastinal lymphoma at age thirty-one. Suddenly, doing makeup for runway shows, the red carpet, and television shows took a back seat to medical waiting rooms, medications, and all of their physical side effects. The celebrities would have to wait.

Shortly before my thirty-second birthday, I was told by my doctor that the pain in my shoulder was caused by the tumor in my chest. I had non-Hodgkin's lymphoma. The idea that I had cancer seemed especially far-fetched since I led a relatively healthy lifestyle: I had never smoked or used drugs, I exercised regularly, worked hard, ate well.

Initially, the physical changes were subtle, but as my cancer treatments progressed, their physical side effects became more apparent. When I first lost my hair to chemotherapy, I pretty much took it in stride. I was working in the fashion industry, and most people assumed that a shaved head was simply my latest incarnation. However, even though I had gotten used to my new look and could not change it, as time passed it began to bother me. My bald head began to symbolize only one thing to me: I had cancer. Taken with all the weird things going on in my body—the bloating (I greatly reduced my exercise routines with the onset of cancer—a mistake), the dark circles around my eyes, the sparse eyebrows, and the pasty complexion—I was left feeling extremely unattractive. And all this coexisted with extreme fatigue and occasional nausea. Not a pretty package.

Eventually, when I still had two months to go in treatment, the salon where I was working fired me, saying, "You are not the pretty boy we hired." I was devastated at the time because although I knew my health was going to be fine, I wondered who would hire me while I was still a cancer patient. As it turned out, I became self-employed. Within a year the makeup line I developed was in stores, launching at almost the precise time that the salon that fired me went out of business. Today I own my own spa as well, so things worked out beautifully. I often think I should have named my spa Karma instead of RAMYSPA. It just goes to show you the power of a positive attitude.

Even though I had a positive outlook, I knew this diagnosis would test my optimism to its limit. In truth, I rationalized that my appearance was not so bad. I was mistaken because the physical changes were gradual. In hindsight, I know that the changes were dramatic. This was evidenced by the fact that I lost my job as the makeup director at a top salon. And the reactions from my loved ones hit home when I visited my parents one weekend. I had been feeling pretty good, but I didn't realize how swollen my face was from the steroids I had been taking during chemotherapy. My mom always put on a brave face and a smile, but I noticed her disappearance from the living room for a while. I found her crying in the kitchen. This was one of my defining moments as I recognized the immense emotional impact a person's physical appearance can have. This event set me into action. I knew that if I felt good, I had to convey that by showing my best face to the world. I needed people to feel as positive about me as I felt about myself. Ultimately, this quest for makeup techniques that countered the effects of treatment would also help others.

A large percentage of cancer patients continue working, going to school, and caring for their families while undergoing chemotherapy or radiation treatments. But you might be suffering the side effects of treatments and feel too frightened, embarrassed, or self-conscious to function at your full potential. I'm here to change that for you. I'll show you how easy it is to disguise the physical evidence of cancer treatments and boost your self-confidence. The American Cancer Society sponsors a program called Look Good, Feel Better in which cancer patients are treated to a day of beauty at top salons where hair and makeup stylists donate their services. The philosophy behind that program is the embodiment of beauty therapy. By making the most of yourself, as a person living with cancer you can regain some control in your life and feel good in the process. In fact, high self-esteem and a positive attitude play a major role in the healing process—and no person who has cancer should have to wear the evidence of it.

The tips you will find here are designed specifically to be effective during times of stress when you are not just busy but also tired and not inclined to spend a great deal of time in front of the mirror. You still want and need to face the world while looking your best. At the risk of sounding sexist, as bad as I sometimes felt about my appearance when I was going through treatment, I believe it is significantly worse for a woman because of the pressures and expectations thrust upon women in our society to look a certain way. Advertisers and the media perpetuate the beauty myth that if a woman can be taller, blonder, thinner, only then will she reach her beauty potential.

This creates a tough battlefield for all women, let alone women living with the side effects of cancer treatments. So it is extremely important to me to emphasize that beauty therapy is not about teaching you how to look perfect during cancer but rather how to help you look and feel like you did before cancer interrupted your life. My goal is to give you the power to simply and easily conceal the side effects of your treatments in order to diminish self-consciousness and embarrassment. I want you to feel downright fabulous.

As you go through your treatments, you will occasionally run into neighbors or acquaintances who are unaware of your situation. As they say hello they may look at you quizzically, wondering, Is she sick? What does she have? Should I say something? Is it fatal? Has she lost her mind or just her hair? As outspoken as I was about my situation, those moments, always bothered me.

I am a strong advocate of self-acceptance. Though we are raised admiring what we think is physical perfection as dictated to us in films, television, magazines, and Madison Avenue, I think the recent cycle in society is to embrace those things that make us different. However, while we are becoming a melting pot of different ethnicities and physical attributes, we are still running out and having our hair straightened, our noses tweaked, debating the virtues of low-carb diets. So we are talking the talk, but I think society is not yet walking the walk. I say we need to truly embrace the bump on our nose, the curly hair and those few extra pounds. The point is to love yourself regardless. This extends to loving yourself while undergoing cancer treatments. You expect your family and friends to love you as you face these challenges, but the most important person whose support you need when undergoing treatment is *you*.

I think some people fear that perhaps their loved ones will not love them if they have an illness or are experiencing physical side effects of treatment. This is a legitimate fear. No one does a happy dance when discovering that a loved one has cancer. The bottom line is that your attitude, your confidence level, and your mindset will affect the reactions of those around you.

Your positive attitude can greatly improve your quality of life and help you to feel your best. Having an illness is not something that anyone plans. It comes as a shock. Everyone who has ever been diagnosed with cancer would agree that they were shocked when they first heard the news. Your survival depends on how you adjust to this surprising turn in the road.

Taking care of a loved one during this time takes its toll on caregivers, who often experience the same emotional turmoil as the person they are taking care of. Therefore, it is very important that you take time out for yourself. Make sure your caregivers don't neglect their own health and well-being. You all need to take care of yourselves. Make sure to watch your caregivers for signs of stress, too. There is no reason why you can't treat a caregiver to a free makeover or a shopping excursion or even a stroll in the park. The key is to take action and make time for each other, which will help make the recovery process less traumatic. You may even manage to have some fun.

As I have given makeup lessons over the years to people living with cancer, I have noticed that they either have a positive attitude or are struggling to overcome the depression associated with illness. Often, a friend or a client tells me that someone close to them has been diagnosed with cancer and that they would like to send this person to me for a makeup consultation. Sometimes, people are too anxious or depressed to even entertain the idea of having a makeup lesson; other times, they embrace the idea eagerly. Individuals come around to addressing the physical side effects of their illness or treatment when they are personally ready. Those people who do come around to taking action are the ones who have the best outcome.

Cancer patients with a positive attitude are in warrior mode. They have made a decision to battle their disease by any and all means possible. This means traditional treatments, possibly holistic treatments, and emotional healing as well. That is where the makeup comes in, because when you look in the mirror and like what you see, it can truly be empowering.

The things that people say to me after having a makeup lesson never cease to amaze me. One beautiful woman in midtreatment came in for a makeup session and brought her sister along for moral support. When we were done, the sister took me aside and thanked me, telling me it was the first time she had seen a glimpse of her sister's bubbly personality in the six months since she had been diagnosed.

When I was just coming out of treatment, I went to work for myself and was very excited about starting my makeup line and having my health back. People kept telling me that I had a glow about me, that there was something special about the energy I exuded. I honestly thought I would have this spark—this wonderful Zen type of quality—for the rest of my life, but the reality is that day-to-day life can kick the Zen right out of you. I went back to my normal, pre-cancer self, being impatient while waiting for elevators, having business headaches and personal dramas. But every time I taught a beauty class for other people living with cancer, I would float home with that same Zen feeling and glow that I experienced posttreatment, thanks to the wonderful energy and gratitude of the women attending my class and the beautiful things they would say to me at the end of each class.

At this same time, as I was recovering posttreatment, two of my mother's dearest friends were diagnosed with cancer. Paula was diagnosed with colon cancer and immediately went into warrior mode, learning everything she could about treatment and her options. I knew she was going to be fine, and thankfully today she is doing great.

My mom's other friend Evelyn was diagnosed with lung cancer and was devastated. She refused to see her friends and basically gave up on life. My mom asked me to visit her in hopes of inspiring her with my positive attitude. I had just launched my makeup line, and I brought her some lipsticks and a blush. When we met, it was obvious that she was dying and she spoke about it very frankly. In an effort to help her overcome her sadness, I told her that I believe God does not give you more than you can handle.

She disagreed with me. My heart sank. I was crestfallen and felt ridiculous that I had brought her makeup as a gift. A few days later, Evelyn called to thank me, saying that she had applied the products and felt better than she had in a very long time. It made me realize the amazing power one can find in a lipstick.

I am not smug when I say that I've had a positive attitude. Sometimes the illness may be bigger than the person, but the attitude you choose to have during your journey can dictate how positive or negative that journey will be.

One woman who attended my Beauty Master Class at CancerCare told me she was diagnosed with breast cancer two weeks after losing her husband to 9/11. She said that everyone kept telling her there is a lesson to be learned in this terrible adversity, but she had no idea what that lesson could be. I had heard similar sentiments from other people with cancer. It can strike the most evolved, well-rounded person who does not necessarily need a wake-up call or life lesson. Sometimes we simply do not see the lesson while we are living it. Sometimes we can only see it in hindsight.

People tend to speak about faith during times of adversity, often turning (or returning) to religion. I always remind them that it is easy to have faith when everything is wonderful. Faith is truly tested in times of adversity, because those are the times when it is the most difficult to have faith. That is what faith is.

When my doctor told me I had cancer, my first question was, "Am I going to lose my hair?" Dr. Moskovitz laughed and said, "You know, most people want to know if their diagnosis is life-threatening," and I replied, "Yeah, yeah, just tell me about the hair."

I had instantly made a decision that I was going to get through this. I was fortunate that my diagnosis matched my attitude.

Most of us have heard it all of our lives: "Beauty comes from within." But what does it really mean? If this statement were true, why do supermodels look like . . . well, supermodels, and the rest of us do not?

I can tell you that the models who reach the top of their field are usually extremely nice, professional, and enthusiastic about their work. I have seen many models who disappeared into obscurity even though they were as physically gorgeous as Cindy Crawford, Claudia Schiffer, and Christy Turlington. They had prima donna attitudes or were in some way difficult. They may have been born with the physical attributes of a supermodel, but they lacked charm, confidence, intelligence, or charisma. They lacked inner beauty.

Inner beauty consists of all the positive qualities of your personality—confidence, strength, compassion. These qualities show up in a person's eyes. We've all met people whom we initially perceive to be beautiful until we spend some time with them. Conversely, we've also met people who don't seem so appealing at first until we get to know them.

When you are first diagnosed with cancer, it is absolutely normal to go through a period of anger and sadness, even if you have always been a very centered person with a healthy dose of your own inner beauty. But as you come to terms with your diagnosis, you can let those destructive feelings consume you or you can take charge of them. When faced with adversity, we have a choice: we can become angry at the world or decide to turn our lemons into lemonade. The anger you feel cannot and should not be suppressed, but it can be redirected and used constructively. Remember, you are angry at the cancer, not at the world.

Spirituality, religion, and faith are important in all aspects of our lives. As a cancer patient, having candles lit for you, keeping crystals, and having friends of different faiths pray for you are all wonderful, especially if they make you feel better. But following traditional treatments and listening to your doctor are equally if not more important. Remember, a healthy body is a beautiful body.

When I was undergoing chemotherapy, an elderly woman named Shelly was receiving hers at the same time. The nurse introduced us, telling Shelly that I was a makeup artist. Shelly pulled off her glasses and asked me what I thought of her makeup. It was perfect, and I told her so. She told me that she was seventy-eight years old, had been battling leukemia for the past nine years, had five great-grandchildren, and was continuing to work forty hours a week as a secretary. She also explained she had "three gentleman callers, and honey, I'm still knocking 'em dead." If this isn't inner beauty, I don't know what is. The point is that beauty therapy is not just about your outward physical appearance, it's also about your inner beauty—your attitude, emotional state, and confidence.

After I had completed my rounds of chemotherapy, I had to have radiation therapy to prevent recurrence of the cancer. I had lived across the street from NYU Medical Center, where my primary oncologist, the brilliant Dr. Tibor Moskovitz, practices and where I received chemotherapy. My routine was to roll out of bed and stop by for chemo on my way to work. When it came time to have radiation, however, my health insurance dictated that I had to have my treatments at Beth Israel Hospital, fifteen blocks away. Having been so spoiled by having my chemotherapy directly across the street from my home, I was outraged at having to take the ten-minute walk out of my way—outraged, that is, until I met a man in the Beth Israel waiting room who was also waiting for his radiation each day. Tall and strapping, he was over seventy years old and had lung cancer that had spread to his brain. He was undergoing chemotherapy and radiation at the same time. According to his doctors, his chance of survival was only 20 percent. He traveled two hours in each direction every day to have his treatments. I realized that I needed to shut up and be grateful. This was an epiphany for me, and I believe my own inner beauty was enhanced as a result.

I was about nine years old when my mother was diagnosed with Hodgkin's disease. I remember how afraid we kids were, how nervous about the outcome of her treatments. The family unit was shaken to its core. At the time (twenty-nine years ago), Hodgkin's disease was not as treatable as it is today, and my mother was hospitalized for several months. Children were not allowed to visit, making the situation scarier for my sister and me because our mother was suddenly gone. We could not see for ourselves whether she was really okay.

On my tenth birthday, my parents decided to sneak me into the hospital to visit my mother. She had been undergoing surgeries to remove her spleen and some lymph nodes as well as receiving extreme radiation. While she suffered some hair loss, it was not obvious to my ten-year-old eyes. If she was in any pain or discomfort, she did not show it. All I saw was good old Mom. Having now undergone much more minor radiation therapy myself, I realize what a brave face she put on for me at the time. As I look back, our visit was astonishingly brief. Only now, all these years later, do I realize why.

Before I became a makeup artist, I was a law student. I dropped out of law school after the first year, knowing for certain that I didn't want to be a lawyer, but I was still unsure what path I should take. Every time I spoke to my mother about it, her advice was the same: "Just do something." She would tell me that it did not matter whether I continued to study law, but I should find my career path no matter what it was and stick to it.

I think this philosophy is important to remember. It reminds me not to be passive, not to be a victim, but to take action. The concept behind beauty therapy is not just about addressing the physical aspects of living with cancer but about taking action, which empowers you. The act of even reading this book, much less following its guidelines, is doing something. The key is not to have a victim's mentality. Take charge of your situation, whether it means just reading a book in search of answers, applying a lipstick to boost your mood, or following any of the beauty therapy steps in this book to improve your appearance or your state of mind. The key is to just do something.

One of the most compelling reasons I decided to write this book is that almost every time I discussed my lymphoma with others, they would share their own cancer experience ("I had cancer . . . ." "My husband had cancer . . . " "My daughter is going through the same thing . . ."). It made me realize how frighteningly commonplace it is. So many people have shared their stories about how difficult it was going back to the office after hair loss, going home to a husband after a mastectomy, dating while undergoing treatment. The side effects of cancer treatments often make you feel too frightened, embarrassed, or self-conscious to function at your full potential.

A common thread in all these stories is that everyone, of course, felt physically bad, but they also felt bad about their physical appearance. I walked away from these encounters knowing that the helplessness they had felt about their situations should not extend to the way they felt about their looks.

I began to think how lucky I am to be a makeup artist and to know what to do to make my skin look healthy. I knew what to do when my hair started falling out from the chemotherapy and my eyebrows became sparse. I knew how to hide the really dark circles that developed around my eyes and how to camouflage my pasty complexion. But what about the average person who might be clueless about makeup? Many cancer patients are at a total loss about how to make themselves look their best. How scary must it be for children to suddenly see Mom or Dad with thinning hair or some other side effect of cancer treatment? How worrisome is it for the professional who needs to continue working? Most people with cancer don't know where to begin to repair the damage to their physical appearance.

My makeup tips are very easy to follow. My personal philosophy is *"minimum makeup, maximum impact,"* which appeals to most people, especially those who are not feeling well and do not want to spend a great deal of time getting ready in the morning. I offer a cut-to-the-chase makeup routine that is so fast and effective you will probably continue to use it for years after the cancer is behind you. My makeup and skin care line, which I launched after losing my job during my bout with cancer, is called RAMY beauty therapy. The idea was, and is, to create products that not only make you look good, but have therapeutic qualities as well. While my minimum makeup, maximum impact philosophy is embraced by modern women on the go the world over, it is especially effective during times of stress when you are not just busy, but also tired and not inclined to spend a great deal of time in front of the mirror; however, you still want and need to face the world looking your best.

I hope this book will be uplifting and empowering in its message to you. I want to show you that taking control of your appearance will make your life better. To that end, I've tried to make it a feel-good tool you can pick up when you're at your worst. I share my philosophy and the tricks I applied during treatment when I was in middle of chemotherapy myself. There are great makeup tips along with an array of ideas for pampering yourself. Many of these techniques are used on the famous faces you see in your favorite magazines and on your favorite television shows, and we're not just talking about women's faces. These techniques can also be used by men. They worked for me.

I have had a lot of time to think about beauty and its effect on people. Before I had cancer I thought of beauty in terms of eye color and symmetry of facial features. As I traveled through Cancer Land, I learned that beauty is power.

The millions of dollars spent annually on cosmetic surgery is proof of the power of beauty. It is not often discussed, but the underlying message from the world is that people who are ill are perceived as weak, and in nature's scheme of natural selection, weakness means that you are not as good as the stronger members of your herd. So when you undergo the physical manifestations that occur during cancer treatments, not only are you perceived to be weak, but in many cases, you are weak. Combine this weakness perception with the fact that you may lose the beauty power you had before treatment began, and it's a whole new ball game.

My mother, herself a cancer survivor, gave me the best advice when I was first diagnosed. She said, "Don't get sad, get angry" (at the cancer). I had to fight to beat cancer. My weapons were and still are humor and beauty. My great hope is that this book will help you reclaim the beauty that is within you as well as your power.

—RAMY GAFNI

NEW YORK CITY

# One

## Beauty Therapy
## for Hair Loss

U ntil I actually began to lose my hair, I didn't really believe it would happen. Neither did my friends, some of whom are world-renowned hair stylists. They assured me that my hair was so thick and healthy that surely I would bypass this particular side effect. They were wrong. When I did start to lose my hair, I finally felt like a cancer patient. Once the hair really started to fall out, I made the decision to have a friend at the salon where I worked at the time shave my head. It felt better than postponing the inevitable and having hair all over the house. But how you handle your

*Immediately upon being diagnosed, cut a sample of your hair so that you have the option of matching a wig to your actual hair. If you can, start shopping for a wig while you still have your own hair; it will be easier to match your natural hair color.*

Kyle White,
Celebrity Hair
Colorist

hair loss is ultimately a personal decision. Just be sure you do what works for you, and don't let others dictate their wishes. Make your own choices, carry them out, and enjoy the fact that you are in control of your new appearance.

My decision to simply have a bare head and cover up with caps or hats during cold weather worked for me. When the manager of the salon—a man totally bald himself, by the way, who never thought to cover his own bare head—pulled me aside and suggested that I might want to consider wearing a toupee, I told him that I thought I looked fine. But inwardly I felt the stress and pressure to make my physical appearance look as cancer-free as possible.

Okay, you're thinking, but you're a man. Lots of healthy men are bald. Well, that's true, but contrary to what you might think, many women find that losing their hair isn't as bad as it's cracked up to be. I didn't feel particularly traumatized until my employer made an issue of it. You may not have a choice about whether you lose your hair, but you do have many choices about how you deal with it.

At CancerCare, I encounter many people in various stages of treatment. What I find interesting is how differently everyone reacts to losing their hair. Some prefer to hide bald heads immediately. Others wear their bare heads with pride. One woman, Harriet, went the wig route the first two times she battled cancer, but she finally rebelled and chose not to cover her bald head during her third bout with the disease. She said that she felt liberated in her baldness and that she wanted the world to see and know what it is to live with cancer. Not hiding her bare head made her feel better. The bottom line, though, is do what makes you feel best. Make your own rules. Choose from these options:

1. Wigs

2. Other head coverings—hats, wraps, turbans, and scarves

3. Au naturel

# WIGS

There are almost as many types of wigs and hairpieces available as there are people who need them. Synthetic or natural, store-bought or customized, long or short, straight or curly, blonde, red, black, auburn, or brunette. Most women try to find a wig that most closely resembles their pretreatment hair in style and color. This is sound advice. However, if you are not shy about change, why not find out how the other half lives and go long and blonde, or dark and curly, if that is the opposite of your own hair? Who could ever forget Kim Cattrall as Samantha in her hot pink wig as she went through chemotherapy on the television series *Sex and the City*?

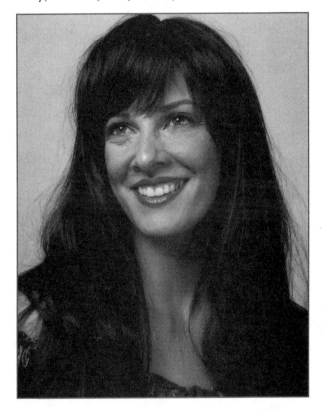

## Types of Wigs

Store-bought synthetic wigs are the most cost-effective, ranging in price from $70 to $200. Human hair and customized wigs are the most expensive, ranging from $200 to $1,200. Human hair wigs are considered the most natural-looking, but I have been astounded by some of the synthetic wigs on the market today. They often look so much like real hair that you would never know otherwise.

Sharon Blynn wearing a long hair, synthetic wig. Wigs can transform your look depending on style, cut, and color.

Depending on the extent of your hair loss, you may even want to consider a hairpiece. The cost $35 to $95 and are great if you have some thinning in your hair but have not experienced complete hair loss. A hairpiece can make the hair you have appear fuller. It is very easy to use. Simply clip it onto your own hair and style as you wish. Hairpieces are often used by celebrities and divas for special events.

# Choosing A Wig

*Wigs often look unnatural because they are too thick or not cut properly. Have your wig cut and styled so you look just as you did before treatment.*

*—Oscar Biandi, celebrity hairstylist*

Depending on your budget, choose either a synthetic or a human-hair wig. Either option can look extremely natural. A wig can feel too warm, like a hat, or itchy. So inquire about the type of mesh used in the wig and about how well it will allow your skin to breathe. The mesh is the material that makes up the cap of the wig to secure the hair to your head. The hair is attached to the mesh. The mesh material is important because it will determine how comfortable the wig will be to wear.

If your goal is to look like you did before you began treatment, choose a color and a style as close to your own hair as possible. I find that erring on the side of choosing a lighter color than your own tends to look more natural than a color that is a tad too dark. However, if you are feeling adventurous, why not try colors and styles that are different from your own? After all, putting on a wig requires less time than cutting, coloring, and styling your own hair.

I have met women who discovered wigs during treatment and liked them so much that they continued wearing them long after their own hair grew back. If you think about it, a wig can be a great quick fix if you don't have time to style your own hair. Each wig is designed with a basic style, but, as with real hair, the styling variations you can achieve are limitless. Take some time to play around with your style and find what works for you or suits your mood for different situations.

## Tips For Buying And Wearing Wigs

Most people will not know you are wearing a wig if you follow these simple steps. They will just think you look good.

- Call the best salon in your city or ask your stylist where the best wigs are sold in your area.

- Decide what type of wig you are going to buy. Synthetic wigs are more affordable, but they cannot be color treated. You can color human-hair wigs.

- Buy your wig extra long so that you can have it cut/wear it in more than one style.

- Ask your current stylist if he or she styles wigs. (You need an honest answer.) Prepare a list of questions that make you feel comfortable and confident. For example, questions about fit, style, color, upkeep or concerns about wearing the wig at the gym, etc.

- Make sure your wig is cut (at least the final cut) while you are wearing it.

- Try to match your actual hair type. For example, if your natural hair is curly, choose a curly wig.

- Request a private room when choosing wigs to avoid the discomfort of trying them on with an audience.

- Ask questions about maintenance, cleaning, and wearing a wig correctly, including the possibility of shaving your head. Ask the salon if package deals are offered for wig maintenance.

## How To Wear/Attach A Wig

Feeling secure is your primary goal, so consult with a wig expert or hairstylist to discover what style or type of wig will work best for you. If you have sensitive skin as a result of chemotherapy or radiation, medically approved double-sided tape or glue adhesives may help alleviate problems. You can also clip the wig to your own natural hair if you have only partial hair loss.

## Styling Your Wig

Louis Licari, the celebrity hair colorist, offers this advice:

> Synthetic wigs cannot be color treated at all, and only certain natural-hair wigs can be color treated. Dark-haired wigs cannot be lightened, and only certain lighter-colored wigs can be changed. So when selecting a wig, always try to match your own color as closely as possible. A wig that is too thick will look like a wig, as opposed to real hair. When it comes to selecting a wig, less is more. A wig that looks skimpy on the stand will look the most natural when on your head.

# Cleaning And Caring For
# Your Natural Or Synthetic Wig

Wigs should be washed or cleaned periodically, depending on how often they are worn. Follow these instructions to keep your wig clean.

- Comb through your wig with a wide-tooth comb.

- Add shampoo to the sink and fill with cold water.

- Let your wig soak for five minutes.

- Gently swish the wig in the soapy water to loosen and wash dirt out. (Always handle your wig gently, because when a wig loses hair, it doesn't grow back!)

- Rinse the wig gently in cold water while holding it in a straight, upright position until thoroughly rinsed. Rinse the hair from the top of the scalp, working down to the tips so that the hair will not get tangled.

- Add regular hair conditioner and work through with your fingertips. (Some wig manufacturers make shampoo and conditioners specifically for wigs, but regular shampoo and conditioners work just as well.)

- Rinse downward thoroughly with cold water.

- Gently blot the wig with a towel. Do not squeeze or wring out the wig.

- Allow to air-dry on a wig stand. Do Not use a hair dryer.

- Comb the wig only when it is completely dry. While the wig is on its stand, use a wide-tooth comb and comb from the bottom, working your way up to the scalp. Combing from the bottom prevents tangling, snagging, and breakage.

- Store your wig on its wig stand and away from direct sources of heat.

# HEAD COVERINGS
# HATS, WRAPS, AND TURBANS

## Hats

Depending on how long or short your hair is and the season, your hat options are practically endless. Even if you never considered yourself a hat person, there's a style for every head, every season, every event. There is a myriad of different fabrics and styles to choose from.

Think of a hat as an opportunity to express your style and personality, not just as a tool to cover hair loss. Hats are great for many reasons. You can spend as little or as much as you want. You can be as casual or as formal as you need to be. You can have an entire hat wardrobe that can add fun and variety to your life.

Hats can be worn over wigs or instead of wigs. They can camouflage a hairless head or flatter thin locks. There are big, floppy straw hats, baseball caps, fishermen's hats, golf hats, berets, close-fitting cloches, knit caps, woolen ski caps (you can wear a scarf underneath these if the wool itches your scalp), brimmed hats with ear flaps that tie under the chin. The choice is yours. Hats are always a great option for protection against the elements as well as being a fashion statement.

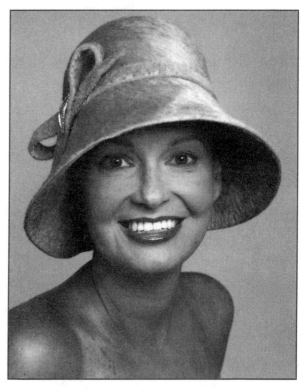

Tracey Pleva Hill, stunning in a hat with a brim that's ideal for concealing hair loss.

## Wraps

Some say a head wrap is more comfortable alternative to a wig. Like a hat, a head wrap (bandana, scarf, handkerchief, or any other cloth you choose) can change and accentuate any look or style. When selecting a head wrap, opt for cotton or cotton-blend materials, because silk and polyester are more likely to slip off your head, and they don't offer the same breathability as cotton fabrics. You can stylize or personalize your head wraps by using ribbon(s), big, funky flowers, a great brooch, or other fun jewelry. Since bandannas come in so many colors and prints these days, you're sure to find one that suits your style.

## Basic Head-Wrapping Techniques

### Variation I

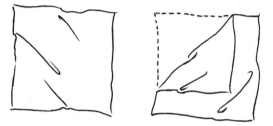

1. Lay the scarf face down. Fold the scarf into a triangle, leaving one point slightly longer than the other.

2. Drape the scarf over your head with the shorter side on top and the points in the back. Position the scarf two or three inches above your eyebrows.

3. Tie the scarf ends in a half knot behind your head. Anchor the flap beneath the knot.

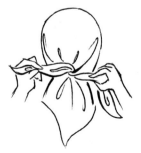
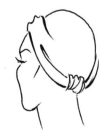
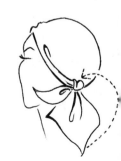

## Variation II

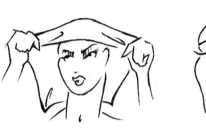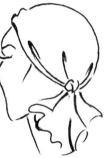

1. Perform steps 1, 2, and 3 of Variation I.

2. Using both hands, spread the lower flap out under the half knot. Spread the scarf down as close to the back of your ears as possible. If you are experiencing hair loss, this will help to conceal it.

3. Bring the flap up over the knot and tuck in the flap and loose ends securely behind the knot.

## Variation III:

1. Follow steps 1, 2, and 3 of Variation I.

2. Select a second scarf in a different fabric, color, or pattern.

3. Twist the second scarf into a rope or braid.

4. Wrap the braid over the basic head wrap and tie it in a half knot at the back or side of your head.

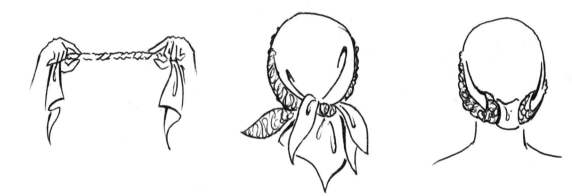

You can purchase prewrapped scarves, turbans, and bandannas, or you can wrap your scarf once and pin it in place with safety pins or decorative pins. This way it can easily be worn or removed like a hat.

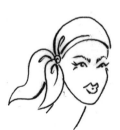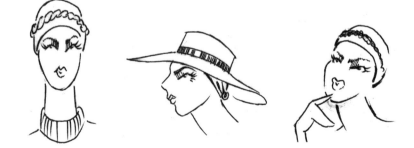

## Turbans

Lana Turner, Elizabeth Taylor, Greta Garbo, Ava Gardner, Marilyn Monroe—these Holly-wood lovelies were the epitome of glamour, chic, beauty, and sophistication. And at some point in each of their careers, they wore turbans and looked fantastic. Turbans or head wraps can be worn with style in any setting (work, play, formal evening, etc.), and they are great time-savers. You can find a variety of preformed turbans at many department stores, accessory boutiques, and hat shops.

## FOR MEN

A hat can totally define a man's style. Cowboy hat, anyone? Think of Colin Farrell and the knit caps he never seems to be without. They not only conceal a bad hair day, they make him look hip. Choose a style that exemplifies who you are and is comfortable. If you have always wanted a hat like Indiana Jones, now's your chance.

Bandannas for men offer many options. You can choose Nascar or Harley Davidson prints, channel your inner biker dude, or make a statement with a solid-colored bandana that matches your shirt or necktie.

## AU NATUREL

Many people choose to just go bare-headed when they lose their hair to cancer treatments. Some wear it as a badge of honor; others are simply not into wigs and have the confidence to show their baldness. Sharon Blynn, pictured on the cover, chose to embrace her baldness. This excerpt from her article, "How I Lost My Hair and Found Myself," exemplifies how most of us feel when we lose our hair as a result of chemotherapy or radiation treatments.

> I had long hair for nearly my entire life. I couldn't imagine cutting my hair, *ever*. Suddenly diagnosed with ovarian cancer, I decided to turn my fear into a positive, empowering choice to reinvent myself. Phase One: cut hair short, donate locks to "Wigs for Kids." When the day came, smiling with nervous anticipation, I tied my hair into ponytails. Two

quick snips and my long hair was gone and I burst into a teary-eyed smile. My dread was overshadowed, banished, by this loving gift. There was much more to come (out, that is) nine days later.

The surreal part of this process began. I would wake up with mounds of hair on my pillow. When I ran my fingers through my hair, large clumps appeared in my palms. I stared at them, feeling helpless. The worst was washing it. Finally, a mere head nod extricating a mutinous cascade of hair brought on Phase Two of my transformation: the electric razor. I sat down, took a deeeeeep breath: Whirrrrrrrrr.

No turning back, I was a bald chick. As I embraced my own chemo-induced baldness with a sense of adventure, I was truly shocked by the overwhelmingly positive response I received.

I gained a profound revelation about my own power, beauty, and femininity. I feel more beautiful, more sexy, more ME than ever.

To read more, go to www.Baldisbeautiful.org

## How To Care For A Bald Head

The skin on your scalp is part of your complexion and deserves the same care and attention as your face.

- Shave off fuzzy new hair growth. The fuzzies just make you look like you are either in treatment or have really bad hair.

- Choose a finish. Apply a satinizing moisturizer for a satin finish, an anti-shine powder for a matte finish, or shea butter (a rich butter extracted from the nut of a shea tree) for shine.

- Use the same cleanser or gentle soap on your scalp as you do on your face.

- Use sunscreen. Choose SPF 20 or higher, since your scalp has never been this exposed to the sun before and is much more likely to burn.

## No-Hair Options for Men

My experience both personally and professionally tells me that many men are more concerned about having and keeping their hair than women. We have all seen the horrific comb-over or toupee that fools no one. But, in fact, a shaved head on a man not only looks contemporary, it more often than not looks downright sexy. Still, when baldness comes with an illness attached to it, it's a double whammy.

Though a hair piece is an option for men during treatment, it is not my favorite option. It's interesting how a wig or hairpiece can help a woman's appearance, but on a man it looks like—well—a man camouflaging a bald head with a hairpiece. I say embrace your bald head, enjoy the freedom of not having to mess with your hair, and choose a cool finish for your scalp, a hot-looking hat, or both.

## How to Wear a Bald Head with Panache

When I was bald, I got many compliments. To this day, many of my friends tell me I looked better without hair and that I should shave my head. Of course, now it's my choice, and I choose to keep my hair for as long as I can. It is comforting to know, however, that if and when my hair thins out, I can shave it and look great.

If your hair is merely thinning, keep it short. Shorter hair looks like fuller hair. But if you can see your scalp through your thinning hair from across the room, it is far more attractive to just shave your head and be done with it.

The best part of being bald is that it is amazingly low-maintenance. Your scalp basically becomes an extension of your face. When you wash your face, simply lather up your scalp with the same cleanser. Use an exfoliating facial scrub on your head, too. The same holds true with moisturizer, bronzer, and so on.

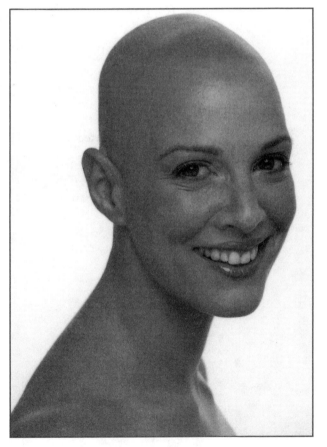

Sharon Blynn, Modeling a bald head with lots of panache!

It's also important to apply sunblock to your head and ears before you go outdoors. You don't realize how much your hair protects you from the elements until it's gone. You are more susceptible to sunburn when your hair is not there to protect you. Windburn, too, for those of you with convertibles. (I learned this the hard way.) And in cold weather, you will learn how warm your hair used to keep you, so wear a knit cap to makeup for lost hair.

Some guys like shine, and buff or wax their scalp to emphasize it. Others prefer not to shine and to have a nice matte finish. For a matte finish, apply an anti-shine lotion or some translucent powder. Yes, powder is a makeup, but if you use translucent (no color) powder, no one will know you have it on. Your friends will only know that they can't check their reflection on your forehead.

## Grow It Where You Can

Men have an option that women don't. We can always grow a beard. I grew a goatee when I lost my scalp hair. It added balance to my face and gave me a whole new look. I would shave the beard off and grow it back periodically during my treatments. It was great having hair to play with.

# Two

## Beauty Therapy Skin Care

The skin is the largest organ in the body. The skin also advertises the state of our general health. Cancer therapies change the texture and condition of your skin. Increased oiliness, dryness, pigmentation, increased or decreased facial hair, and inflammation are all possible side effects. You will probably discover that your favorite skin care products no longer work as well as they once did. The reverse is also true: products that never seemed to do the trick can suddenly work wonders. The point is that cancer therapy brings about changes in the skin.

In this chapter, you'll learn how to put on a healthy, glowing complexion to mask looking pale and tired. You'll also learn the best ways to revitalize your skin. Think of this as an opportunity to permanently revitalize your complexion and learn some tricks for keeping your skin looking healthy and glowing. You may also find, like me, that one of the very few positive side effects of chemotherapy is the absence of pimples and blemishes. However, be aware that the hue of your skin may change during treatment. On the days immediately following chemo, you may appear very pale or even yellow, and occasionally you may even look a little gray. Even as a professional makeup artist, I must admit I did not always notice these color changes in myself, possibly because, it is difficult to be objective about your own appearance. So read on and learn how to conceal what you do not want the world to see and how to accentuate the positive.

## SKIN CARE PRODUCTS

My philosophy is that your skin's needs change every day. One day your skin may feel dry and require moisturizer, another day you may feel oily and can skip the moisturizer, and yet other days you may need moisturizer only on certain parts of your face. Only you can evaluate what your skin needs on a particular day.

Using certain products can actually make the difference between you looking like a cancer patient and looking like someone with fabulous skin. The following paragraphs discuss the active ingredients that you should look for in your cleansers and moisturizers to keep your skin exfoliated, healthy, and youthfully glowing. In the interest of simplifying your skin care routine, look for products that combine several qualities. For example, choose a moisturizer or a liquid bronzer that contains fruit extracts or antioxidant vitamins to revitalize your complexion as you moisturize. Or choose a bronzed-tone blush that can color your cheeks and do double duty as a bronzer. You can also find a cleanser that contains glycolic or salicylic acids and has a scrubbing texture.

• ALPHA- OR BETA- HYDROXY ACID Fruit acids gently exfoliate, ridding skin of the dull surface layer of dead cells. As a result, fine lines are diminished and a rosy glow to the complexion is imparted. Alpha-hydroxy products can cause mild irritation to sensitive skin, but I find it to be an almost miracle cure for a pale or lifeless complexion. If your skin is indeed sensitive, choose a formula that has 2 percent Alpha-hydroxy or less, and use it only every other day. This allows your skin to regenerate and helps guard your complexion from irritation.

- SALICYLIC ACID Salicylic acid is found in many skin care products that are used to treat blemished skin. Salicylic acid products can be drying, so they are best for an oily complexion. Products containing salicylic acid really help to clear the complexion and bring a little color to the surface. You can try a gel or cream formula. The average strength of salicylic acid in acne-fighting products is 2 percent, but opt for 1 percent if you have excessively dry or sensitive skin.

- GLYCOLIC ACID Glycolic acid products are similar to alpha-hydroxy products but stronger. They are generally used for people who want to smooth their complexion and diminish fine lines. Check the percentage of the acid in the product before buying it. Ten percent glycolic acid is very strong. Six percent is ideal for most people, and anything lower is not very effective except on very sensitive skin.

Whether or not you use products with active ingredients, there are several essential skin care products that will help maintain healthy skin and give your complexion an instant visual boost.

- FACIAL SCRUBS Used once a week, scrubs are a wonderful way to slough away dead skin and get the blood circulating. I always used the scrub on my scalp during my hair-loss period. Many scrubs contain beta- or alpha-hydroxy acids, salicylic acid, and skin renewing antioxidant vitamins such as vitamins A and C. If you have sensitive skin and would like to exfoliate in a gentler way, choose a facial scrub with soothing ingredients such as chamomile or cucumber. It should have round scrubbing beads such as jojoba instead of jagged ones. Another option for sensitive skin is an exfoliating mask that removes the dead surface skin by adhering to it as the mask dries. Then you simply rinse off the mask and can avoid the harsher method of scrubbing altogether.

*The most important beauty ritual for me is not the ritual itself but time. Taking time for myself is the ultimate luxury.*

Sarah Brown, beauty director, *Vogue*

- MOISTURIZERS Even if you do not think your skin needs to be revitalized, a good basic moisturizer should always be part of your routine. It is one simple step that can smooth your complexion and body as well as protect it. Applying moisturizer after a shower or bath helps to lock in the moisture. If you are not inclined to reapply moisturizer throughout the day, make sure you apply it (hand or foot cream, facial and body moisturizer) at night before going to sleep. This way your products are working for you instead of the other way around.

- TINTED MOISTURIZER These products are great for simultaneously moisturizing and adding color to your skin. Tinted moisturizers are particularly good if you do not like wearing foundation or bronzer. You should look for one that contains sunscreen, moisturizes, and has a reflective quality, which diminishes the appearance of fine lines and gives the illusion of a smoother complexion. Choosing a color that is one or two shades darker than your skin tone will do double duty as a bronzer.

# COLOR

- BLUSH The right color can really bring your face to life. Blush can be more subtle than bronzer. If you are extremely pale, choose a pale pink blush. If your skin has some color, choose a blush that has a bit of brown in it. It can be rosy or tawny, but it should not look too blue. Brown-based colors will always look more like your own natural glow. The best test for blush is to apply the color to your eyes. If it does not look good on your eyes, then it is not the right color for the rest of your face, either.

- HIGHLIGHTER This can be used on the eyes, cheekbones, and around the lips to magically bring life and light to your face. It is available in powder, shadow, cream, stick, and pencil form. When applied on the eyelids and under the arch of your eyebrow, highlighter will bring them forward and make you look more awake. When applied high up on your cheekbones, highlighter will emphasize your bone structure. Applied to the center of your lower lip, highlighter will make your lips look fuller. A photographer's trick is to apply highlighter to the Cupid's bow of your top lip and on your chin just under the center of your lower lip in order to make your lips look fuller and more luscious. Choose a highlighter in a neutral or pale color. Pale pink or white will work beautifully on any skin tone and can look the most dramatic; yellow or gold tones are much more subtle if you are more conservative but still want to use a highlighter. Either way, you can control how dramatic or subtle the effect will be depending on how much highlighter you apply and how well you blend it. Stick formulas offer the most control, followed by cream. Loose powder highlighter offers the least control.

- BRONZER Skin care products aside, if all else fails and you simply want to add a needed glow to your complexion, bronzer is the way to go. It is available in powder, gel, stick, or cream form in a variety of colors that can take you from a healthy glow to a deep tan. Whether you choose a powder, gel, or liquid bronzer, simply apply it wherever the sun would naturally give you color. The key is to select the correct color and blend it well. Bronzer is also a great way to extend a spray-on tan or is a fine alternative to spray tanning, especially if your goal is to control how much color you end up with or if you want less of a tanning commitment.

- SELF-TANNER The new self-tanning gels and lotions really look natural and no longer impart the dreaded orangey color. Be sure to exfoliate your skin first to avoid a splotchy application and so that your tan will fade evenly. The great thing about self-tanning is that you are not damaging your skin as you would by baking under the hot sun or using a tanning bed in order to achieve a beautiful tan glow. Self-tanning has the added bonus of lasting for three days and not washing off like a bronzer.

## BASIC SKIN CARE
## REGIMEN FOR THE FACE

If you do not follow a particular skin care regimen because you feel overwhelmed by all the different options, let me simplify the process with this basic, but essential routine.

CLEANSE YOUR FACE Choose any basic facial cleanser. Look for products labeled for sensitive skin. Avoid basic bar soap, since it can strip the skin of its essential oils and be drying. If prone to blemishes,

*When I just cannot fight the fight, I find washing my face and starting over is the best way to transform a bad day.*

Lori Bergamotto, senior beauty editor, *Lucky* magazine

choose a cleansing pad with salicylic acid. Use cleansing pads in a pinch when really busy or traveling. If you are in a hurry or feel too tired to properly wash your face, use a premoistened baby wipe or cleansing sheet for a quick cleanup.

MOISTURIZE During the day, use a moisturizer that contains sunblock. At night, use either a basic moisturizer without sun protection or a heavier moisturizer indicated for nighttime use to treat and condition your skin while you sleep.

# COMBATING THE EFFECTS OF CHEMO AND RADIATION

In order to take good care of your complexion during cancer treatment, it is important that you understand the side effects of these treatments. By understanding the physical manifestations, you will be better able to assess and care for your skin.

Some types of chemotherapeutic agents cause changes in the skin, hair, and nails. These effects may include but are not limited to hair loss; darkening of the skin, hair, and nails; increased sensitivity to sunlight; itching; and nonspecific skin rashes.

Radiation therapy can lead to acute and chronic changes in the skin being treated. Short-term changes include redness, swelling, and even blistering. Long-term skin changes are hyperpigmentation (darkening) and thinning of the skin, leading to chronic redness and the appearance of many little blood vessels.

Everyone reacts differently. You may not have any side effects, or you may have some or all of them in varying degrees.

Chemotherapy and/or radiation therapy are immunosuppressants; therefore, they make your skin much more susceptible to bacterial, viral, and fungal infections. Be vigilant about keeping your skin clean and free of irritants. It is important to consult your physician at the first sign of infection. It is also important that you take precautions so as not to further irritate skin already sensitized by treatment. Here's how:

- *Limit sun exposure and avoid sunburn*: Sun exposure even after completion of radiation therapy should always be avoided because of the increased risk of developing skin cancers at the irradiated sites.

- *Avoid cosmetics and moisturizers that contain exfoliants:* These products include alpha-or beta-hydroxy acids, glycolic acids, and salicylic acids that can irritate already sensitive skin. Protect the affected area from rubbing and scratching.

- *Use only water to clean the affected skin*: After washing, try using aloe vera–containing lotions to soothe the skin between radiation treatments.

## Beauty Therapy For Dry, Chafed, Or Flaky Skin

1. Use a moisturizing cleanser and/or a cleanser for sensitive skin. A gentle baby wash is ideal.

2. Switch to an alpha-hydroxy or retinol (vitamin A) moisturizer, especially at night. This may initially cause the skin to flake even more for a day or two. If this happens or if your skin is feeling very sensitive, choose a gentle moisturizer that does not contain fruit acids or vitamin A.

3. Use a gentle exfoliating scrub once or twice a week. If any redness or itchiness occurs, it could be a sign that you are irritating your skin by overexfoliating, so only use the alpha-hydroxy moisturizer every other night and the exfoliating scrub once every five to seven days.

4. Cut down on your intake of caffeine, which acts as a diuretic, and increase your water (not soda, fruit punch, or sports drinks) intake.

## Beauty Therapy for Oily, Blemished, Acne-Prone Skin

1. Use a gel cleanser, which works best for reducing oil.

2. Follow with an astringent, preferably one that contains salicylic acid, which is excellent for drying pimples and exfoliating the skin.

3. Use an oil-free moisturizer, only on the areas you feel are dry.

4. Apply a salicylic acid clear gel made to clean pores and dry blemishes at night or just keep your face bare. Sometimes when you overly strip your skin in an effort to reduce oiliness, your oil glands produce even more oil. Dot a little of the gel on minor blemishes, let it dry, then rinse it off. This way you won't get it on areas of your face that don't need it.

## Beauty Therapy for Dark Under-Eye Circles

1. Apply one of the new under-eye treatments created to diminish dark circles. The antioxidant vitamins (particularly vitamin K) in these products help to constrict the blood vessels under the skin (with regular use), thereby diminishing the dark circles. Look for an eye moisturizer that also offers a very subtle shimmer to reflect light and conceal dark circles instantly.

2. Apply a moisturizing concealer that is one shade lighter than your skin tone all around the entire eye area, including the lash line to the brow bone as well as directly below your lower lash line, because the dark and red circles extend above the eyes as well as below. Blend. Apply concealer around the entire eye not only to bring your eyes forward and give them a lift but also as a primer for any eye makeup you apply later.

3. Apply highlighter or shimmer to the eyelid and the inner corner of the eye. Blend.

4. If you have prominent dark circles and feel that you need additional help, it is time for a diversionary tactic. After following steps 1, 2, and 3, apply a dark eyeliner and mascara to the upper lash line only. Then when people look at you, their eyes are naturally drawn upward to the liner and mascara and away from the dark circles underneath.

# BASIC SKIN CARE
# REGIMEN FOR THE BODY

## Relieving the Red, Itchy Skin of Radiation Therapy

The sunburn-like redness, itchiness, and sensitivity to the skin in the area where the radiation is focused can become a problem. Even a minor dose of radiation can make your skin sensitive to the touch while making it appear light pink to a deeper red in color, like a sunburn. It is very important to recognize that your skin type and the duration of your treatment determine the way your skin responds to radiation so that you know how to combat potential problems or even prevent them from happening. This is not the time to use body scrubs, salt scrubs, alpha-hydroxy cleansers, or products with salicylic or glycolic acids, alcohol, or vitamins A or C on or around your affected area.

### *Beauty Therapy During Radiation Treatment*

1. Cleanse with a very soft shower sponge when bathing because you do not want to irritate your skin. Be particularly gentle around your affected (radiated) area.

2. Use gentle liquid moisturizing cleansers such as those made with soothing oils—for example, Dr. Bonner's All In One liquid cleanser.

## Beauty Therapy After Radiation Treatment

1. Apply a light coating of 100 percent pure aloe vera gel to the affected area to moisturize and cool. Trust me, this feels great.

2. Continue with the gentle cleansing approach you used during treatment with the addition of a sunscreen with a minimum SPF 15 that offers protection for both UVA and UVB rays. Look for sunblock with broad-spectrum protection.

## Reducing or Eliminating Scars

Polymer silicone sheets are now available over the counter at your local drugstore. Applied daily, they significantly reduce hypertrophic and keloid scars resulting from surgical incisions.

# Three
## Makeup as
## Beauty Therapy

I always say the most important beauty tool is an open mind. Even if you didn't wear makeup before, now is the time to experience the difference makeup can make in your life. When you apply it correctly, people notice you, not the makeup. What's more, you need not wear a full face of makeup in order to conceal the side effects of cancer treatments. Simply employing one or two of the tricks of the trade that you'll learn in this chapter will make a difference. For example, did you know that just wearing concealer and/or mascara alone can make you look more rested and bright-eyed?

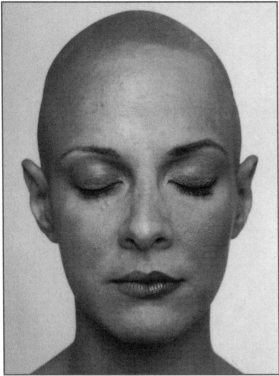

Sharon Blynn with only one side of her face enhanced with makeup. This is a combination of the Two and Five Minute routine. Customize to find the best routine to address your needs.

If you're thinking that you're not the makeup type and the thought of applying it is making you feel overwhelmed, don't panic. I am simply presenting all the options. Choose a routine that suits you best, whether it means employing the classic face routine or simply wearing only a bronzer.

## THE SIMPLE EQUATION FOR BEAUTY

Beauty is not complicated—it takes only a very simple equation to create beauty. The equation consists of playing down your less attractive features and playing up your most attractive features. It's as simple as not applying a lipstick just because it is handy but instead taking a moment to choose a flattering color. It amazes me that some people spend more time selecting shoes than lipstick. The fact is that whether you are a world-renowned actress, a supermodel, a bank teller in Arizona, a homemaker in Kansas, or a lobbyist in Washington, the game plan remains the same: In order to look your best, emphasize your best features to draw attention away from less flattering ones. If wearing a full face of makeup (foundation, concealer, powder, eye makeup, blush, lipstick) has always been a part of your daily routine, now is the time to simplify your life by eliminating unnecessary steps and learning new makeup techniques that are more effective and faster.

Men needn't be afraid of makeup. The key is to apply it so that it doesn't look like you're wearing makeup. So if you're a guy, trust me: makeup will help you look good. The photos of me in the color insert of this book were taken when I was the makeup artist on a photo shoot. At the time, I was midway through chemotherapy and had started using makeup tricks to hide my sallow skin and to look glowing and healthy. In these pictures, I am wearing bronzer all over my face and neck to rid my skin of its pale, sallow coloring. I applied concealer all around my eyes (on my eyelids as well as up to my brow bone) to hide the very dark circles I had at the time. I put clear mascara on my upper lash line to emphasize the few eyelashes I had left; light brown/taupe powder shadow on my eyebrows, as they were near disappearing; a subtle shimmer on my eyelids to further bring the eyes forward; and lip balm. The point here is that I didn't look as if I was wearing makeup—I just looked good. Here's how to achieve this look yourself.

## BASIC MAKEUP TOOLS

Proper makeup application requires the right tools. Never skimp on cheap brushes. They don't work as well and they don't last. If you already have a good set of makeup brushes, you're ahead of the game. If you have cheap ones, now is the time to upgrade. Below is a list of the tools you will need. These are the same types I use for makeup applications at the spa, photo shoots, and runway shows. If you don't want or can't afford to invest in all of them, buy the ones marked with an asterisk.

- blender brush
- blush brush*
- bronzing brush
- brow brush
- concealer brush
- cotton balls
- eye contour brush
- eye definer brush*
- eyelash curler
- eyeliner brush*
- eye shader brush

- eye shadow brush

- latex sponges

- lip brush

- powder brush

- tweezers*

## MAKEUP OPTIONS

Cancer treatments are as individualized as our physical reactions to them, so you can easily customize your makeup routine to suit your special needs. It doesn't matter if your goal is to minimize the appearance of eyebrow or eyelash loss or to simplify your makeup routine. The end result should make you look terrific. For example, you can follow the fast and easy two minute face routine in Chapter 4, adding the solution for sparse eyebrows if necessary. This makeup routine only takes three or four minutes with a bit of practice—a minimum investment of time that will help you look and feel terrific. Check out the other routines, too. There is one to fit every need, skin type, color, and nationality.

You may find that your skin type will change. If you have been oily all your life, your complexion may be dry, during treatment, or vice versa. So don't insist on sticking with your precancer foundation if it no longer works well on your skin. It is important to feel secure and comfortable in your own skin. But just because you look fine without makeup doesn't mean you couldn't look better with it. Applying a bit of tinted moisturizer or lip balm could be your entire makeup routine. The key is to keep an open mind and do what makes you feel your best because when you feel your best, you look your best. As you go through cancer treatments, you're sure to have some days when you feel (and maybe look) just awful. So put on that lip gloss and look in the mirror. I guarantee that what you see will lift your spirits.

# WARM OR COOLS— WHICH ONE ARE YOU?

Warm colors look more yellow or orange. Cool colors look more blue or pink. Every cosmetic color has undertones of both warm and cool hues but will look predominantly warm or cool when applied. Everyone looks better in warm colors where foundation or concealer are concerned. When adding color to your look (blush, eye makeup, lip color) you probably look better in cool tones if you are very fair. Look for colors that appear more pink or blue as opposed to warmer tones like browns, coppers, or gold, which look great on medium and darker complexions.

If you are not sure whether you should be wearing warm or cool colors, try combining them. Warm shades are flattering on most people, but cool colors sometimes look too blue or obvious. Combining both warm and cool colors ensures that you will look good because they will balance each other out. For example, if you are wearing a warm-colored blush, sweep a bit of a cool-colored blush on top of the warm color or on the apples of your cheeks. For women of color and for Indian and Asian women, all the suggestions and tips I offer in this book hold true for you, too. I have a very universal approach to beauty. The key is finding a concealer or foundation that matches your personal skin tone. Unlike the colors you wear on your eyes, cheeks, or lips, concealer and foundation should appear invisible against your complexion. Everything else—all the color suggestions you will read—will work on any skin tone. If your skin is dark, opt for a darker brown shadow or pencil. Otherwise, you should not focus on the color suggestions but rather on the makeup application techniques that I share with you.

# MAKEUP 101—FOUNDATION

Foundation can literally be the foundation to your makeup routine. It creates a flawless canvas for your makeup application, hides imperfections, and helps your makeup stay put. Some people are blessed with a flawless complexion and can skip foundation. The rest of us with blemishes, discoloration, uneven skin tones, and redness need foundation to create the illusion of a perfect complexion.

## Selecting the Perfect Color

Foundations are available in liquids, creams, powders, sticks and tinted moisturizers. Foundation should always match your skin tone exactly. Everyone has a myriad of different undertones in their complexion—yellow, blue, red, orange, pink. Yellow-based foundations work best on most skin types. Pink-based foundations just look pink. The most common mistake I see in makeup applications is when someone wants to add a little color by using a foundation that is darker than her skin tone. It doesn't work and only succeeds in giving a mask-like or ashen look to the face. A foundation that is too light can also end up looking mask-like.

If you want to find your correct foundation color, apply a drop of foundation on your jawline and blend it in a circular motion with your fingertips. Wait one minute for it to dry. Like paint, foundation color changes slightly when dry. The correct color will be invisible on your skin.

## Selecting the Perfect Foundation

Don't panic when you see foundations in every conceivable form: liquid, cream, powder, stick, and tinted moisturizer. Here's what each does.

- LIQUID FOUNDATION Available in light to heavy coverage, liquid foundation works best on skin that is dry or has fine lines and wrinkles, because it imparts the smoothest finish. A silicone-based formula is ideal for combination skin or to create the illusion of a smoother complexion, because the silicone glides over fine lines instead of getting into the nooks and crannies of the skin's texture. Oil-based formulas are good for dry skin and water-based liquid foundation is good for oily complexions.

- DUAL-FINISH CREAM TO POWDER FOUNDATIONS These foundations offer light coverage (but more coverage than traditional powders) for all skin types. People who do not like liquid foundation but want to even out their skin tone usually love dual-finish foundations because they can be easily applied with a sponge or puff and are packaged in convenient compacts just like translucent powders.

- STICK FOUNDATION Sticks offer medium to heavy coverage for all skin types. Stick foundation can be your best makeup tool if you want one product that is multipurpose and easy to use. The stick formula is more dense than liquid and dual-finish foundations, so it can double as your concealer.

- TINTED MOISTURIZER This formula offers the lightest coverage. It is basically moisturizer with a hint of color. Tinted moisturizer will not make much difference if you are looking to correct an uneven complexion, but it can add a touch of color to an otherwise listless complexion. If you would not even entertain the idea of wearing foundation, then a tinted moisturizer can be considered a multipurpose product for you—moisture and a bit of color in one.

## Applying Foundation

You have selected the correct color base, so you're halfway there. Now you need to know how to apply your foundation correctly to achieve the look of a flawless complexion as opposed to a made-up look.

- LIQUID FOUNDATION Foundation need not be applied all over the entire face; it can be applied only where you need it. For example, if you have redness around the nose and chin areas, apply foundation only on those spots.

   1. Apply a dot of the foundation where needed on your face, or apply it on the five points of your face: a dot on each cheek, the chin, the nose and the forehead.

   2. Blend it into your skin using your fingertips.

- DUAL FINISH CREAM TO POWDER Available usually in compact form, it is often considered easier to use than liquid foundation. Apply with a sponge where needed and blend. It dries to a powder finish.

   1. Dab foundation where desired on your face.

2. Blend with a sponge. This works well because the sponge absorbs the excess foundation, leaving you with a more natural finish. If you desire heavier coverage, blend with your fingers.

- STICK FOUNDATION Stick foundation is best applied only where you need it (as opposed to all over the entire face).

   1. Apply stick foundation around the entire eye area.

   2. Apply on other areas of your face where your skin tone needs evening out (often around the nostrils and chin, for example).

   3. Blend with your fingers or a sponge.

   4. Some stick foundations dry to a powder finish. If the one you are using does not, then set with powder.

- TINTED MOISTURIZER Just apply as you would any moisturizer by blending it in with your fingers.

# BRONZER

The best product you can use to achieve a look of good health and vitality is a bronzer. A bronzer is not to be confused with a self-tanner, because this product gives you a healthy, sun-kissed glow until you wash it off at day's end. A self-tanner, in contrast, gets darker after several hours and lasts for several days.

## Types of Bronzers

POWDER BRONZER Powder bronzer is best for oily skin.

GEL BRONZER Gel bronzer is best for combination skin.

LIQUID BRONZER Liquid bronzer is best for dry skin.

Of the different types of bronzers on the market (gel, liquid, powder), my favorite is the gel. It can easily be applied and blended like a moisturizer. Powder formulas are also a good option, but powder can sometimes oxidize as the skin's natural oils come out and cause the color to intensify.

## Selecting the Best Shade of Bronzer

If you are naturally very pale and use foundation colors such as ivory or bisque, select the lightest shade of bronzer available, since a little bit of color on fair skin goes a long way. If your complexion is dark, using a dark bronzer gives skin a more vibrant tone. If in doubt, the surest bet is to choose a medium bronzer. You can layer on the color depending on your skin color.

## Applying Bronzer

To apply a bronzer, simply blend it in wherever the sun would naturally give you color. Bronzer can be applied alone on bare skin or on top of your makeup.

- POWDER FORMULA Use a bronzing or blush brush and sweep the bronzer across your cheekbones, over eyelids, and along your hairline. Then apply the bronzer along the jawline, blending downward to bronze your neck.

- LIQUID OR GEL FORMULA Use your fingers and apply a dot of bronzer to each cheek, tip of your nose, forehead, and chin, then blend. Follow by adding a dot to each side of your neck and blend upward.

# CONCEALER

If you walk away from this book having learned only one thing, it should be that concealer is your friend. Supermodel Cindy Crawford has been quoted as saying that if she could have one beauty product on a desert island, it would be concealer. Concealer hides your secrets from the world. It makes you look rested, even if you aren't. It camouflages dark circles and redness.

## Selecting the Perfect Concealer

Look for a concealer with as many active ingredients as possible. Rose extract, for example, reduces puffiness; antioxidant vitamins A and C help to diminish fine lines around the eye area; and vitamin K is purported to reduce dark circles with regular use.

Concealer is available in a variety of shades. A yellow-based color one shade lighter than your skin tone or foundation usually works best, but don't go any lighter than one shade or you'll end up with the reverse raccoon effect. Concealer hides the dark circles that often occur during chemotherapy and the sleeplessness associated with some medications.

## Selecting the Perfect Formula

- STICK CONCEALER Stick formula offers the heaviest coverage. If you have lines or wrinkles around the eyes, be careful with stick concealer because it will crease up and draw attention to those things you want to downplay.

- CREAM (POT) CONCEALER Creams offer medium to heavy coverage. Like the stick variety, cream concealer can be heavy and must be applied carefully with a brush. Cream concealer can also be a bit dry. If it is, I mix it with a little eye moisturizer.

- LIQUID CONCEALER Liquid concealer offers light to medium coverage and is available in a wand, tube, or flow-through pen. Liquid concealer gives the lightest and smoothest finish and so is best if you want to avoid the cakiness often associated with heavier concealers.

## Applying Concealer

Concealer is applied around the entire eye area. Dot along the lower lash line and over the eyelid, remembering to apply on the inner eye area. Blend with a sponge or your fingers. If the concealer seems too heavy to apply to your eyelid, then it is not the correct formula for you.

Remember that the darkest area is usually just where your inner eye meets the bridge of your nose. Applying coverage there makes the most dramatic difference. Concealer can also be used on other areas of the face where needed.

# POWDER

Powder is necessary in order to set your foundation and concealer. I prefer a powder that is completely translucent. Most modern formulas are translucent, meaning that they are more finely milled so that skin color can show through. Truly translucent powder, offers no color, looks white in the packaging, and is completely invisible on the skin. It works on any skin tone and does not alter the color of the skin, concealer, or foundation. Translucent powder is also the great equalizer. If makeup appears too dark or intense, the powder will subdue it, and it works equally well on eyebrow filler, eye shadow, and blush.

## Selecting a Powder

- PRESSED POWDER This is my preference because it helps avoid that overpowdered look. There is less powder on the brush or puff than with loose powder, and therefore less powder gets applied to the skin.

- LOOSE POWDER Loose offers more coverage than pressed powder and is a favorite of makeup artists. For home use, stick with pressed powder. It will give you the best results and is easiest to apply.

## Applying Powder

Once concealer and foundation are applied and blended with a sponge or your fingertips, dip a powder brush or powder puff in the loose or pressed powder, shake off or tap off excess, and sweep over your face and eyes. You want to use just enough to set the foundation and concealer and keep your makeup in place. I often hear women say that their blush (or eye shadow) slides right off their face. Powder prevents this from happening. Contrary to popular myth, your face does not absorb the color like a sponge, but without powder the makeup has nothing to which to adhere.

# EYE MAKEUP

Once you have applied foundation, concealer, and powder, you have prepared the canvas on which you will now add color to bring out your features and create the art that is your face. For many people, the eyes are their best feature; for others, making up the eyes correctly makes the eyes their best feature. The eyes classically require more makeup steps than the rest of the face, but if made up properly, they can project your best face to the world.

## Eye Shadows

Eye shadows contour and enhance eye shape. They can be used to create depth or bring deep-set eyes forward. The correct color eye shadow can enhance your eye color, make small eyes look bigger, and make close-set eyes look wider apart.

### Selecting an Eye Shadow

- POWDER EYE SHADOW The most common formula, powder shadows can be layered and blended easily with an eye shadow brush. They are available in matte and shimmer formulas.

- CREAM EYE SHADOW Cream shadows can be applied with a brush or with your fingertips. They are fast and easy to apply. They're available in matte, shimmer, and cream gel formulas.

### Applying Eye Shadow

You can choose any myriad of ways to apply eye shadow. Any formula can be applied either as a sheer wash of color from the lash line to the brow bone or as a contour, in which case a lighter color is used on the eyelid and under the brow bone and a deeper shade on the crease of the eye.

## EyeLiner

The real key to achieving great-looking eyes with no (or sparse) eyelashes is eyeliner. Eyeliner creates the illusion of a full row of eyelashes. If you have no eyelashes at all, mascara is obviously useless, but eyeliner can create a natural-looking lash line.

## Selecting an Eyeliner

- SHADOW (CAKE OR POWDER) EYELINER Shadow liner is my preference. It is applied with a wet eyeliner brush, it wears beautifully, and it creates a soft, flattering line. Shadow liner looks like a real lash line.

- PENCIL EYELINER Pencil eyeliner is a favorite of many women because they find it easiest to use. Choose a pencil that is not too soft, not too hard, and blends smoothly.

- LIQUID EYELINER Many people find liquid eyeliner difficult to apply, especially when using a brush. Many cosmetic companies offer liquid liner in a pen, which can be easier to apply. I find, however, that liquid eyeliner sometimes looks harsh like a dried paint line and not at all natural.

- GEL EYELINER Like shadow liner, gel liner is applied with an eyeliner brush and is long-lasting. Gel liner is a great solution if your eyelids are oily or if your eyes have a tendency to tear.

## Applying Eyeliner

1. Using the liner of your choice, dot or make a line as close to the roots of your upper lash line as possible, extending slightly past the outer lash line. Using a cotton swab or latex applicator, blend or smudge the line a little to soften it.

2. Apply dark brown or black mascara to your top lashes only.

3. If you have no eyelashes at all, go over the liner with an eye shadow one shade lighter than the liner. This will soften the line as well as add texture and dimension to more fully create the look of eyelashes.

4. You can repeat steps 1, 2, and 3 on the outer, lower lash line. However, I seldom recommend mascara for anyone's lower lashes, as it visually drags the eye down and draws attention to dark

*I like to do something with my eyes. The eyes are the windows to the soul. So when my eyes are looking good, I feel like everything looks better.*

Denise Rich, founder of the Angel Network

circles, bags, lines, and wrinkles. If you're having trouble with dark under-eye circles, you can skip lining the lower lash line so that the weight of the eye will be on the upper lash line, thereby visually lifting the eye and giving you a clean, less made-up look.

# MASCARA

## Selecting a Mascara

Select a water-resistant mascara formulated for sensitive eyes and be sure to remove your mascara every night with eye-makeup remover (the makeup removing pads are fast and easy) or facial cleanser. It is also best to avoid trendy colors like purple or burgundy if your objective is to look natural, and stick to black and brown shades. If you dislike the "look" of mascara but need to enhance your eye lashes, choose a clear mascara that lengthens and thickens without that mascara look.

There are several types of mascara to choose from: water resistant, waterproof, and long wearing tints.

- WATER RESISTANT  This is the formula I recommend most highly. It has staying power, but comes off easily with makeup remover or facial cleanser without the need for harsh rubbing.

- WATERPROOF MASCARA  Often preferred because it stays put when your eyes tear. I do not recommend waterproof mascara for use during treatment because it is difficult to remove and excessive rubbing can cause even more eyelash loss.

- LONG WEARING TINTS  Long wearing tints stay on your lashes for two to three days and like waterproof formulas, they are difficult to remove. For this reason I do not recommend using this formula during treatment because leaving mascara on lashes for several days can inhibit new growth and may even cause existing lashes to fall out.

## Applying Mascara

1. Apply mascara to your upper lash line only. This will "lift" your eye. Not applying mascara to the lower lash also alleviates any chance of mascara running and drawing attention to fine lines or

bags around the eyes. If you feel your eyes lack definition without mascara on your lower lash line then apply eye liner on your lower lash line instead.

2. To apply mascara hold the wand as close to the roots of your eyelashes as possible. As you pull the wand from the base of your lashes to your lash tips, "jiggle" the wand back and forth, left to right, to help fully coat each lash. Add an extra coat to the outer half of your upper lash line for every decade over thirty years old (as we age, our eye lashes get shorter).

A SPECIAL NOTE: Once mascara is used, it develops bacteria in about three months, so to help prevent causing an eye infection, it's very important to replace your mascara every three months, even if it was only used once.

## Making Your Eyes Look Their Best

Here is my step-by-step guide for bringing out the best in your eyes. This version is perfect when you have extra time or desire a more dramatic look.

### *Classic Eye Makeup Routine*

1. Apply concealer all around the eye area and set with translucent powder.

2. Using an eye shadow brush, sweep a pale, golden shadow all over the eye area from the lash line to the brow bone.

3. Using an eye contour brush or the edge of your eye shadow brush, apply a taupe, sable, or brown eye shadow to the outer crease of your eye. Blend.

4. Using an eye definer brush, apply the same color shadow used in step 2 to the lower lash line to define your eye shape.

5. Wet the eyeliner brush and line the upper lash line with chocolate, mahogany or brown liner.

6. Apply dark brown or black mascara to your upper lashes only to really lift and open up your eyes.

7. Choose an eyebrow pencil, powder, or pomade that is one shade lighter than your hair color to fill in your eyebrows. Brush through.

Here is my tried and true shortcut if you're in a rush or just don't have much energy.

## Quickie Eye Makeup Routine

1. Apply concealer all around the eye area and set with translucent powder.

2. Apply dark brown or mahogany eyeliner to the upper lash line. Use either a pencil or a gel or powder formula with an eyeliner brush. If an eyeliner brush is too much of a hassle, just use an eyeliner pencil. Apply the pencil as close to the base of your eyelashes as possible so that you get a fine line. If you feel you cannot make the line look smooth or symmetrical, use a small brush or cotton swab to smudge the line and make it look smoky. A smoky line need not be perfect to look good.

3. Apply mascara to your upper lashes only. Mascara and eyeliner applied to upper lash line will instantly lift and define your eyes.

4. Add color to your eyelids by either sweeping blush over your eyes with a blush brush or drawing on color with a multiple-use stick and blending it with your finger, or simply use your finger to apply a face gloss, shimmer, or cream blush to the lids.

## Preventing Makeup from Running

Going through a health crisis is not easy and you may find that your emotions are often very close to the surface. If your emotional state is so fragile that you often find yourself teary, here are some pointers for avoiding running makeup.

• Apply mascara and eyeliner to the upper lash line only. This will not only give your eyes a lift but will reduce makeup from running down your cheeks.

- Opt for a water-resistant mascara as opposed to a water proof mascara, which can dry out and damage eyelashes.

- A pencil or gel eyeliner will stay on longer than a powder. If you prefer a powder or cake eyeliner, as I do, then add a gel or pencil liner on top of the powder eyeliner.

- Avoid powder eye shadows, which make a bigger mess if you cry or tear profusely. Opt for a cream or shimmer color on your eyes, or if you prefer powder, try sweeping a light-colored blush over your eyes with a blush brush.

- Keep a foundation stick or concealer with you. Apply it where needed around your eye area or face after a tearful episode to clean up makeup and to freshen your appearance.

*On those mornings when I wake up looking and feeling disgusting, I go out to eat with friends. They get me away from focusing on my own stuff and always get me to laugh.*

Jane Pratt, editor-in-chief of *Jane* magazine

# BLUSH

If applied properly, blush will give you a warm, healthy glow. The old school of makeup required blush to be the equivalent of hot-pink racing stripes. The modern approach is to forget about contouring and go for a subtle, natural-looking color.

## Selecting the Best Blush

Blush is available in a variety of formulas and textures. There's an easy trick to finding the right blush color for your complexion. Using a blush brush, sweep the blush over your eyes. If it doesn't look good, then it's not the right color for you. If it looks flattering on your eyes and highlights your eye color, then you've found the perfect blush color for the rest of your face.

## Types of Blush

- POWDER BLUSH Blush in a powder formula is the traditional favorite, and it's best applied with an angled blush brush. All powder blushes are not created equal. The best formula has the finest powder granules (micronized) and is silicone treated for the smoothest, most even application and the longest wear.

- CREAM OR GEL BLUSH Available in a pot or a tube, cream or gel blush is fast and easy. A cream formula is great for dry complexions and a gel formula is best for those with an oily complexion. Many of these products can be used on the eyes and lips as well.

- BLUSH STICK Blush sticks are a wonderful fast and portable option. A blush stick can be a cream, gel, shimmer, or stain formula. Many blush sticks are formulated for multiple use, meaning they can be used on the eyes and lips as well as the cheeks.

- BLUSH STAINS Blush stains are primarily liquids that can be applied with a spatula, sponge, roller-ball applicator, or as a stick. The general complaint is that the stain sets too quickly. If not immediately blended, you are left with a dot of color on your cheeks like Raggedy Ann. Stains are wonderful on the lips, however, imparting a rosy shot of color that lasts all day. One of my favorite tricks is to apply a blush stain to the lips, then reapply lip balm over it as needed. You'll look like you have lipstick on all day long.

## Applying Blush

One of the most common questions I'm asked is exactly where blush should be applied. My foolproof method is to look in a mirror, smile, and apply blush from the apples of the cheek up into the hairline (outside of the eye area). I also like to apply a little blush along the hairline using the blush brush to make the color look a little more natural, then sweep a bit over the eyes as well. Applying the blush along the hairline makes the color blend in with your own skin color. By applying the color elsewhere on your face, you pull the whole look together. If your goal is a very rosy or flushed look, then apply a pink blush or rosy cheek stain to the apples of your cheeks.

A true professional makeup trick is to contour the cheeks by applying a nude, tawny or otherwise subtle color from the apples of the cheeks, blending upward to the hairline, then smile and apply the pink blush just to the apples of the cheeks for a pop of color.

The most flattering blush color is very warm and golden but with a hint of rosiness that looks almost like a light bronzer. Blush can also be used to further conceal dark circles and under-eye bags. Simply sweep a bit of powder blush above the cheeks, just under your eyes.

- POWDER BLUSH Apply powder blush with an angled brush as opposed to a flat brush. An angled blush brush follows the contours of your face, so it offers easier and more natural-looking application. If you want to use the blush as an eye color as well, simply sweep the blush over your eyelids using a blush brush.

- CREAM OR GEL BLUSH Simply dab the cream or gel blush onto the apple of your cheek and blend with your fingertips along the cheekbone.

- BLUSH STICK Use the stick to draw some color onto your cheeks and blend with your fingertips or a sponge. If your blush stick is formulated for use on the eyes or lips, draw the color onto your eyelid or the crease of your eye and blend with your finger. A blush stick can be applied directly to the lips like a giant lipstick.

## LIP COLOR

I believe people can and should change their lip color with the season or with their mood. Lipsticks come in a seemingly endless array of colors and formulas. We all have a friend who has found a favorite color and formula and will stock up on it as though that lipstick were canned food and they were being loaded into a bomb shelter.

If you find a lipstick that works extremely well for you, that is wonderful, but most of the world is on the eternal search for that delicious, elusive, perfect lipstick. When I asked women about their favorite beauty ritual when having a bad day, many told me that buying a new lipstick is their favorite inexpensive and fun, pick-me-up.

## Types of Lipsticks

- CREAM FORMULA This is the classic wax-based formula. Many luscious ingredients (jojoba oil, avocado oil, or vitamin E, for example) are added to cream formulas to make them more moisturizing and conditioning than ever before.

- SHIMMER FORMULA Elementally the same as the cream formulas, shimmers are great for adding that little touch of frosty shine. Shimmer formulas are the most long-lasting, because even if the color fades or is eaten off, a shimmery pearlescent residue remains.

- SHEER FORMULA Sheer lipsticks are the most moisturizing but the least long-wearing. Sheer formulas are great if you have dry lips or aren't used to wearing lipstick, but you want to try adding a little lightweight lip color.

- MATTE FORMULA Matte formulas are long-wearing, but they can be very drying. They have always been my least favorite because I think dry-looking lips are unappealing.

- LONG-WEARING LIP COLOR These new revolutionary formulas do last all day, but they are extremely drying and require a glossy topcoat to be reapplied throughout the day. You might as well just reapply a standard lipstick that won't dry out your lips.

- LIP BALM The un-lipstick. Lip balm with color does not give the same color impact as a lipstick, but it is a terrific conditioning alternative. Lip balm is especially appealing if you don't care for lipstick, but you want a polished look.

- LIP PENCIL Lip pencils are most commonly used to outline the lips to define them and give lip color a more finished appearance while preventing color from bleeding. Lip pencil can also be used on its own as a long-wearing lip color. Either line and fill the lips with a pencil or (my preference) apply lipstick first, then outline and fill in your lips with the lip pencil. This is the more moisturizing option, since pencil alone can sometimes be drying. Additionally, you can apply more lipstick after the pencil for more moisture and color.

• LIP GLOSS Lip gloss is a great addition or alternative to lipstick. Simply apply over your favorite lipstick for a glossy shine or wear gloss alone for a quick and easy lipstick alternative. The new opaque lip glosses and liquid lip colors that come in tubes wear well and are often more moisturizing than lipsticks and easier to reapply. Lip glosses come in tubes, wands, flow-through pens, and pots.

## Selecting a Lip Color

Should you wear nudes, corals, reds, or browns? My advice is to forget whatever you've been told by makeup artists, beauty expert, or your mother and try different lipsticks as objectively as you can. Wear the ones that look best.

Remember, your face changes over time, as does makeup. Formulas are constantly being improved upon to feel more lightweight, conditioning, and long-wearing. New colors and textures are developed. So there are no rules. Makeup is not permanent, so play, play, play.

# Four
## Face Time—
## Making Up Your Face

How much time is necessary for a complete makeup routine. There is no single answer. For you it may be simply taking five seconds to apply your lipstick before leaving the house. Or it may be a twenty-minute routine involving foundation, concealer, a couple of eye shadows, mascara, blush and lip gloss. Usually, it is somewhere in between. Contrary to popular myth, not everyone sticks to the same routine every day of their lives. Your beauty routine can fluctuate depending on how much time you have to get ready, how well rested you feel on a given day, whether you want to look professional, sporty or glamorous. It is fine to vary your makeup routine and how much face time you need to achieve the desired effect. This chapter has some different routines ranging from the minimal thirty-second face to the all-out glamour of the classic evening face. I cover different beauty solutions and time constraints to suit any occasion.

You can use these routines and simply add steps to upgrade from one to the next. For example, you can wear the two-minute face during the day and add foundation, eyeliner, and lip pencil to amp up your look to the five-minute face for the evening. These are just guidelines. You can mix and match the steps from the different faces to customize your look.

## CHOOSING YOUR COLORS

In this modern age of beauty where individuality is celebrated, almost anything goes. Gone are the days where your lipstick had to match your blush and your eye shadow had to match your dress.

That said, what is important is how to know if the colors you select are right for you. Trial and error. Go to a makeup counter and play. If you are timid about wearing makeup, go for light, neutral colors. As you become more confident in your makeup, you can add accents of color, such as a bright-colored lipstick or plum eyeliner.

When it comes to figuring out which colors go together well, chances are that if a color looks good on you, it can be worn with another color that also looks good on you. For example, if an eye shadow looks great with your skin tone and enhances your eye color, then wear it with your favorite lipstick.

## THE MINIMALIST: THE THIRTY-SECOND FACE

Even this simplest of routines will make you look more polished and perfected. Any one of the three steps can be used alone in a pinch to make a difference in your appearance and feeling of well-being. The thirty-second face can be applied by even the most novice, klutzy, makeup-intimidated person and yield fabulous, fast results.

1. Apply foundation stick all around the eye area and where needed on your face to perfect your complexion.

2. Apply mascara to your upper lashes only.

3. Apply face gloss or a multiple-use stick to your eyelids, cheeks, and lips, blending the eye and cheek color with your fingers. If you really want to pare down your routine, choose a product in a color that has multiple uses. For example, a light brown pencil can be used to fill in your eyebrows, as an eyeliner, and as a lip liner.

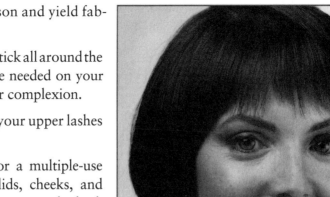

## THE TWO-MINUTE FACE

1. Apply concealer all around the eye area. Blend with your fingers or a sponge.

2. Apply bronzer or tinted moisturizer to your face or blush to your cheeks and eyes.

3. Apply clear or dark brown mascara.

4. Apply a sheer lip gloss or lip balm.

Suzanne Murphy is wearing her own wig and the Two Minute makeup routine. The objective? Look healthy and glowing in two minutes flat!

## THE FIVE-MINUTE FACE

1. Apply foundation to even out your complexion, either all over your face or where needed—around the nose and chin—to make your skin look flawless.

2. Apply concealer all around the eye area, especially at the darkest point of your inner eye area. Blend with your fingers or a sponge.

3. Using a powder brush or puff, set concealer and foundation with pressed powder.

4. Using a blush brush, sweep a warm, neutral blush from the apples of your cheeks up into the hairline, along the forehead, and over the eyelids.

5. Line the upper lash line with chocolate, mahogany, or brown liner.

6. Apply dark brown or black mascara to the top lashes only.

7. Apply lipstick and define your lips with a lip pencil, if desired.

## THE CLASSIC DAY FACE

1. Follow steps 1, 2, and 3 of the five-minute face.

2. Add a light matte eyeshadow from the lashline up to the brow bone. Choose a pale golden or pale pink color.

3. Add a darker-colored eye shadow to the crease of eye and blend well. Then line the lower lash line with the same color. Use a light brown or taupe shadow if you have a fair complexion; rich brown or plum for darker skin tones.

4. Proceed with steps 4 through 7 of the five-minute face.

## THE CLASSIC EVENING FACE

Taking your day face into evening should be the easiest part of your makeup routine. If you have already selected the most classic, flattering colors for your day palette, then it stands to reason that those same colors will work for evening. Just a few simple steps add a little more impact and glamour:

1. Add lip gloss to your lip color. Choose either a clear gloss or a gloss in an opaque color with a subtle shimmer.

2. Enhance your eyeliner. Using the same eyeliner you wear for day, make the line a bit deeper, thicker, and/or extend it a little more past the outer lash line. For the more adventurous, switch to black or apply an eyeliner with a shimmery finish on top of your day eyeliner.

3. Bump up your blush. Add a little more blush to your cheeks and sweep over your eyes with a blush brush.

4. Add a shimmery eye shadow to your eyelid and under the arch of your eyebrow. (Not recommended for more mature skin, as shimmer can draw attention to fine lines.) Adding a pearly highlighter to your eyes, cheeks, lips, and collarbone (yes, your collarbone) over your makeup is a superfast way to take your day look into evening using just one product.

*When I have a lot of work and cannot focus or sit still, I will take a heap of editing or writing and go get my makeup done. It forces me to concentrate—I cannot get out of the seat.*

Dany Levy, creator of dailycandy.com

## CONSOLIDATED BEAUTY

It's a current trend to have eyebrows, eyeliner, lip liner, and even blush permanently tattooed to save time when applying makeup. I'm not a fan of this practice because tattooing is permanent. Remember that your features change with time (you will not wear lip liner the same way at age sixty as you did at age twenty), and cosmetics' colors and formulas change over time as well. There are three ways to keep your look polished without making a lifelong commitment and without overdoing it.

1. Apply concealer all around the eye area and set with a bit of powder. Skip the foundation unless you really need the added coverage.

2. Apply lots of mascara to the upper lash line only. Fun, flirty lashes are always pretty and really do bring out your eyes.

3. Either apply a multiple-use product (available in stick, pot, or compact form) to your eyes, cheeks, and lips or get a small makeup kit that contains the colors you want and need but won't take up a great deal of room.

## MAKEUP FOR EXTREMELY SENSITIVE SKIN

A reaction to cosmetics can be caused by various things. You might be allergic to the fragrance or to the pigment used in certain colors. Many fine brands of cosmetics are now made to be skin-friendly and are ideal for sensitive skin. As a rule, darker, richer colors and colors with a pearl or shimmer tend to cause the most reaction, so opt for lighter matte colors instead. If you have an adverse reaction to cosmetics, don't immediately give up on makeup. Instead, find out why. Have allergy tests done to see what particular ingredient you may be allergic to or simply experiment with other makeup brands and formulations. Start by trying fragrance-free products or products formulated specifically for sensitive skin. I've seen many people have success with mineral-based products, though I don't feel that you need to limit yourself to mineral-based cosmetics only.

Another thing you can do is keep your makeup routine to the bare minimum. The less you apply, the less likely that you will have a reaction. The key is not to give up on the concept of enhancing your features just because you have had an adverse reaction to certain products in the past. Even finding a pencil that you can tolerate to line and define your eyes and lips is better than wearing no makeup at all. But if you who have extremely sensitive eyes and cannot wear any eye makeup whatsoever, wear glasses with color-tinted lenses and play up your lips with a beautiful color. There are many ways to overcome the sensitivity issues. The key is your willingness to try new things to see what works best for you.

## LOOKING LIKE A STAR:

Tara Kraft, the beauty director of Star magazine, has a few simple tricks for creating a star look.

• Brown false lashes applied to the top lashes only and coated with black mascara—look real and very flirtatious.

• A bit of illuminating lotion mixed with foundation will easily give you a star glow and really helps your skin to photograph well.

• White eyeliner in the lower rim of the eyes helps eyes pop.

• Red lips always yield a movie star look.

## Wearing Red

Here's how to have beautiful red lips. This is something that concerns both makeup mavens and women on the go who wear minimal makeup.

• If you are not used to wearing bold lip color, start with a sheer red lipstick or gloss.

• To tone it down, apply a nude lip liner first (a matching red lip liner adds impact), or apply the red lip color over your favorite lipstick. This way, you'll be wearing red while managing to keep it within your comfort zone.

• For all-out red, a lipstick in cream or matte formula is best. Remember to keep the rest of your makeup toned down. One simple look that is striking with red lips is a bit of eyeliner on the upper lash line, mascara, and a well-shaped brow. Go easy on the eye shadow when wearing red lips.

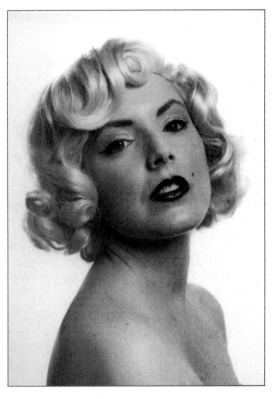

• For thin lips, opt for lighter reds with a subtle shimmer. Choose deeper, darker shades for full lips. Some warm, sheer shades of red work beautifully for everyone.

Deciding which shade of red is right for you depends on your taste, age, and lip shape. There are literally millions of shades and formulas to choose from, and (here's the fun part) it's all about trial and error.

# TRANSITIONING FROM SUMMER TO WINTER

A big part of my makeup philosophy is that when you wear the correct colors and formulas, they should work year-round for both day and evening. But during the autumn and winter months, you should make some minor adjustments to encompass the season's trends.

Suzanne Murphy as Marilyn Monroe. I simply amped up the eyeliner on her upper lash line, added a bolder red lipstick and lip pencil, and added a highlighting shimmer stick to her eyes, cheeks, nose, and shoulders to transform her everyday two-minute makeup into a Hollywood goddess. This illustrates how a few simple steps can create any look to which you aspire.

This is the time of year to wear a more formal finish on your skin. In the hot summer months, it's possible to skip the foundation and apply a less structured look using powder alone. In the fall or winter, a more finished complexion is appropriate and can protect your skin from the elements. While I still suggest using foundation only if you need it, winter is less casual than summer and your complexion should reflect that change. Apply a yellow-based foundation that matches your skin precisely only where needed to even out your complexion.

Richer, stronger lip colors are year-round staples. Burgundy, plum and rich brown are the current rage. My suggestion is to definitely try a richer shade of lip color for the colder months. If darker colors intimidate you, try easing into deeper shades by applying a stronger-colored gloss over your favorite lipstick. Wearing lip gloss gives you the bonus of keeping your lips extra moisturized during colder winter months.

Lastly, a great way to call attention to your eyes without feeling overly made up is to apply a cream shimmer to your eyelid or on your inner eye (on either side of your nose). This makes your eyes sparkle and appear more awake without competing with a stronger lip color.

## SHIMMER AND SHINE
## AT ANY AGE

Words like *shimmer, shine, radiance* and *luminous glow* have recently entered the makeup vocabulary. They describe healthy skin, the very basis for beauty today. Regardless of age, everyone can apply a neutral shimmer cream high up on the cheekbones to play up bone structure or on the eyes or lips to play up those features. Shimmer can also be worn on the collarbone if you wear a lowcut top.

The key is not to apply shimmer cream in an area that has fine lines or wrinkles, since shimmer will only serve to emphasize them. Only teens and twenty-somethings should apply shimmer with a heavy hand. The rest of us should start with a small amount and build gradually to a finish that looks great.

To achieve shine or a dewy finish, use a moisturizing formula foundation and apply powder with a very light hand. Apply a cream gloss or stick formula to your eyes and use a cream or gel blush on your cheeks. Again, if you are not an under-thirty supermodel, choose one feature that you want to shine. Alternate adding shine to your eyes, lips, and skin each time you apply makeup. Remember that the most important shine comes from within.

*It's all about brightening up. I keep a flesh-toned shimmery highlighter and sheer red lip gloss on my desk for manic moments.*

Gwen Flamberg, beauty director, *Fitness* magazine

## AMPING UP YOUR MAKEUP FOR THE HOLIDAYS:

Here are simple steps to add to your makeup routine to turn any look into a festive holiday look. You'll be the belle of the ball. The best part is that you can apply these steps to your favorite makeup routine to add some seasonal spark, or use them for a very fresh-faced holiday look.

1. Apply a dark eyeliner to your upper lash line using a moistened eyeliner brush. Extend the line a bit past your outer lash line and smudge the line a bit for a dramatic smoky effect. (Think modern Audrey Hepburn.)

2. Choose a red lipstick to add instant glamour and holiday spirit. It doesn't have to be a mega-bright opaque lip color (though if you can pull that off, you will definitely be the center of attention). There are shades and formulas of red for anyone and everyone today. Sheer red lipstick might look like bright hooker red in the tube, but it can be incredibly sheer and wearable on your lips. You can apply a sheer, bright red lipstick or gloss on top of your favorite lipstick. This is a great way to rosy up a lip color with which you are already comfortable, especially if wearing all-out red on its own is intimidating for you.

3. Add a neutral shimmer to your eyes, cheeks, lips, and collar bone to light up your skin, brighten and highlight your features, and truly create some holiday magic. Apply a cream or stick formula highlighter (which offers more application control) to your eyelids, focusing on the inner corner of your eyes. Blend with

your fingers. Then, still using your fingers, add the highlighter high up on your cheekbones and just below the center of your lower lip. This will emphasize your cheekbones and give your lip a fuller, poutier look. Finally, rub some of the highlighter onto your collarbone and shoulders to make your skin look luminous and glowing with holiday cheer.

# Five

# Eyebrows and Eyelashes

Shaping your eyebrows is by far one of the easiest ways to make the most dramatic change in your appearance. A well-shaped brow can lift and open up your eyes and make you look younger, more sophisticated, more rested, and healthier. Well-groomed eyebrows make you look fabulous.

If your eyebrows are truly unruly or are just growing back after chemotherapy and you do not know where or how to begin shaping them, your best bet is to have them done once by a professional. Then be diligent about removing new hair growth in order to maintain the shape.

Eyebrows are my specialty, and I have very distinct opinions on how they should be shaped. I am personally against waxing the brows

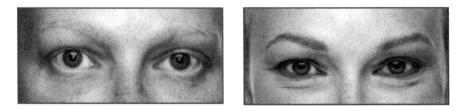

Tracey Pleva Hill before and after filling in her eyebrows with "Miracle Brow" and lining her eyes in order to fill in her lash line.

(waxing is for cars) because there is no precision with waxing, you are removing rows of hair indiscriminately, and waxing is very harsh on the thin, delicate skin around the eye area. Waxing is especially harsh when your skin is more sensitive due to cancer treatments. Threading (a technique that predates tweezers, where thread is used to lasso the hair to be removed) is an option if done by an expert, but my technique of choice is tweezing and trimming, which is easy enough for you to do at home. Here's what you'll need.

- A large mirror, preferably near a bright window. Use a magnifying mirror if your vision demands it.

- A good pair of tweezers, preferably slanted and rounded.

- Small grooming scissors for more control, with a curved shape so that you do not get a hard line when you trim.

- A small brush (a baby toothbrush or an old mascara wand that has been cleaned with makeup remover is ideal).

- Forty minutes set aside so that you do not rush, which often leads to the worst brow fiascos.

- My Miracle Brow, which is like a pencil and a powder melted in a gel base, in case you need to fill your brows. The compact comes in one universal shade that works on any hair color so it's foolproof.

## DETERMINING THE BEST BROW SHAPE

1. When it comes to tweezing eyebrows, less is more. Once you have plucked a hair, it is gone. That being said, begin by objectively looking at your face in a mirror.

2. Be sure to stand two to three feet away from the mirror so that you do not see every little hair. Look at your eyebrows and think about where you may need to remove hair.

3. Determine what the best shape of your eyebrow should be. Your goal should be to enhance the natural shape of your brow. It is usually a mistake to try to copy a model's or celebrity's eyebrow shape from a picture because the shape that works for one person is not necessarily the best for another.

4. To determine exactly where your eyebrow should begin and end, hold up a makeup brush or a pencil vertically against the side of your nose. Where the pencil point or brush tip lands by your brow is where your eyebrow should begin. The eyebrow should end a little past your outer eye so that it frames your eye completely. If it grows too far down your cheeks, it will drag your eyes down visually.

5. To determine where your arch should be, move closer to the mirror and stare straight ahead. A good way to determine where the arch should be is to look at the top of your eyebrow. Directly under the highest point is where your arch should be.

# TWEEZING

Once you have determined the right shape, you're ready to tweeze.

1. Brush your eyebrows upward. If there is much length, trim the excess length with the scissors as conservatively as possible as though you are trimming split ends.

2. Tweeze from underneath your brow, removing one row of hair from the beginning of the brow to the end. Pluck hairs out in the direction of hair growth. If necessary, remove second row of hair from directly underneath your arch to open it up. Then clean the hairs that are not part of your eyebrow or your hairline but exist somewhere in the middle, fuzzying everything up. Lastly, pluck between your eyebrows. Keep in mind that the most common mistake is overplucking, so let common sense be your guide.

3. Using the brush, comb your brows downward. If there is still excess length, trim it, cutting against the grain. Remember to trim very conservatively. You can always cut off more, but once you trim too much, there is nothing to do but wait for the hairs to grow back.

If you follow these simple steps, your brows should look finished and polished, which will open up your whole face and lift your eyes. But mistakes do happen. If you think you have botched up the shape of your eyebrows, the best thing to do is stop. Let your eyebrow hairs grow back for at least three weeks. You might be tempted to pluck strays, but let the hairs grow back as fully as possible instead. This is the fastest way to get great eyebrows again.

# BROW MAKEUP

The good news is that if you suffer partial or complete eyebrow and eyelash loss during treatment, you can camouflage it simply and beautifully with makeup. If possible, take a photo of yourself before your eyebrows start to thin out. This will give you a visual map to follow later when you are filling in your eyebrows with makeup.

## For Sparse Eyebrows

If your eyebrows get sparse during treatment or as they are growing back after chemotherapy, choose a pencil, brush-on brow shadow, or brow pomade one shade lighter than your hair color unless your hair is light blonde or silver, in which case you should select a color that is one shade darker. The most common mistake you can make when filling in your eyebrows is selecting a color that's too dark and not blending the color well. When unsure or in doubt about which color to select, choose light brown or taupe, which will look natural on almost any hair color. Feather the product along your eyebrow (where your eyebrow is or where you would like it to be). Brush through using a spoolly brow brush (it looks like a mascara wand), a small toothbrush, or whatever brush is included with the brow filler you are using. Brushing through the brow filler is very important. This blends the makeup on your eyebrow and removes the excess so that you end up with a fuller and more plush, more natural-looking eyebrow as opposed to a made-up, drawn-on look (remember Joan Crawford?), so blend, blend, blend.

If your eyebrows have become dry and lifeless, apply some hair conditioner to them while you are in the shower, leave the conditioner on for a few minutes, and rinse. You can also apply a leave-in conditioner to them in the morning to help your eyebrows maintain their glory throughout the day.

## For Complete Eyebrow Hair Loss

Opt for an eyebrow filler that comes in a universal shade, meaning a neutral shade that will look natural on any hair color. If you can't find one, choose a pencil and brush-on brow powder, that are both one shade lighter than your hair color.

- If your hair color is blonde or light brown, use a blonde or taupe pencil with a light brown brush-on brow color.

- If your hair is dark brown or black, use a medium brown pencil with a dark-brown brush-on brow color.

- If your hair is red, use an auburn pencil with a light brown brush-on brow color.

### Drawing a Natural-Looking Eyebrow

1. Using the pencil, feather or dot along your brow bone lightly, re-creating the line of your eyebrow.

2. Using a brow brush, apply the shadow (brush-on brow color) over the pencil.

3. Brush through.

These two products used together create a texture and dimension that is incredibly similar to a real eyebrow. If your eyebrows have disappeared altogether and you're not quite certain where your eyebrow line should be, look at the photo of yourself prechemo and attempt to follow that line. If this gets tricky, simply follow your brow bone and try to create a brow line that looks good to you. Also, if adding an eye shadow over the pencil is too cumbersome, simply apply translucent powder with a powder brush or puff over the pencil. This will have the same texturizing effect as eye shadow, but it is much faster—you just sweep the translucent powder over the entire brow and go.

Another option is to use a product I created in response to many of my client's requests for a shortcut to a natural-looking brow. Miracle Brow is like a pencil and powder melted into a gel base. It comes only in one universal shade, so there is no guesswork in selecting the right color, and it has a two-ended brush that makes application very easy. Remember that no one is perfectly symmetrical. Your eyebrows are siblings, not twins. Most of us have one brow that is higher than the other or more arched. This is the human condition. Yes, an experienced brow expert can create the illusion of more symmetry, but try not to obsess about symmetry when creating your brow line.

# RE-CREATING THE LOOK OF FULL AND BEAUTIFUL EYELASHES

If you lose some or all of your eyelashes during treatment, you want the solution to be simple and effective. There are two ways to go here. One is to use makeup to re-create the look of full, healthy eyelashes, such as lining the eyes with a shadow or pencil liner. Another is to use false eyelashes.

## False Eyelashes

False lashes can be cumbersome to apply. For a cancer patient, the adhesive can cause eye irritation. But there might be a time when you really feel the need to use them as you're going through chemotherapy— for example, if you have a big wedding to attend. Check with your doctor, because you may be particularly immunosuppressed as a result of the chemotherapy, which will make you more vulnerable to infection or irritation. If you have your doctor's blessing, go for it. False lashes can give you an instantly glamorous look.

## Types of False Eyelashes

There are two kinds of false eyelashes.

1. Full rows, which add density to the whole lash line. Full lashes are easier to apply, but they do not look as natural as individual lashes. If you've lost your eyelashes entirely, however, these are the way to go.

2. Individual lashes, which can be used to fill in sparse areas or dramatically open up the eye area. Individual lashes require a steadier hand and a bit more practice. They are best for filling in the existing lash line or adding a touch of drama to existing lashes.

## Applying False Eyelashes

1. Before you apply the lashes, line your upper lash line with a mahogany eyeliner and smudge it slightly for a smoky effect. This will help to conceal the lash band and offer you a guideline where to apply the false lashes if you have already lost your own eyelashes.

2. Apply a thin line of adhesive to the lash band on your false eyelashes and give it a moment to become sticky.

3. Apply the false lashes as close to your natural lash line as possible starting at the outer corner of the eye, working your way inward and pressing the lash band gently. Use the eyeliner as a guide.

4. If you still have lashes of your own, apply mascara to blend your lashes in with the false ones. Curl the lashes using an eye lash curler. If you do use an eyelash curler, be extra gentle so as not to pull too aggressively on your natural eyelashes. If you have no eyelashes of your own, then after you apply the false lashes, go over the eyeliner with more eyeliner or with a thin line of eye shadow to blend everything together and conceal the lash band.

# Creating A Great
# Lashline Without False Eyelashes

If you decide to skip the false eyelash routine altogether, you can opt for the much easier and more effective method of applying eyeliner and mascara. See page 66 for choosing and applying the best eyeliner. See page 68 for mascara information.

## Caring for Eyelashes:

Eyelashes may thin out or disappear altogether during chemotherapy. It's best to avoid curling your lashes, as the roots are weak and curling may increase lash loss. If you want to have your lashes tinted, be sure to have it done by an experienced professional who comes highly recommended. While it is illegal in some states, I know many people who have had good results. Lash tinting works best on light hair. It does not look as dramatic or last very long on darker hair. This advice will help you during your recovery period as eyelashes grow back.

1. Curling your lashes on occasion is fine, but you are overdoing it if you see breakage or lash loss. Most makeup artists agree that curling your lashes opens up your eyes and makes them appear larger. I find that most people's eyelashes are already curling in the right direction. For daily care, you can curl your lashes while applying mascara—gently pressing against the lashes with the mascara wand does the trick.

2. Remove mascara and eye makeup religiously every night before bedtime.

3. Once a week, apply petroleum jelly or castor oil to lashes and leave on overnight to soften and condition. Apply with a disposable mascara wand for even distribution.

4. A well-balanced diet can help you grow and maintain fuller lashes.

5. Do not rub your eyes. If you must rub, do it gently so as not to irritate the delicate skin around the eye area or cause eye lash loss.

6. To create the illusion of fuller eyelashes, apply concealer all around the eye area (lash line to brow bone, too) and set with powder. Apply a shadow liner with a moistened eyeliner brush to the upper lash line and smudge the line slightly with the brush. Apply mascara.

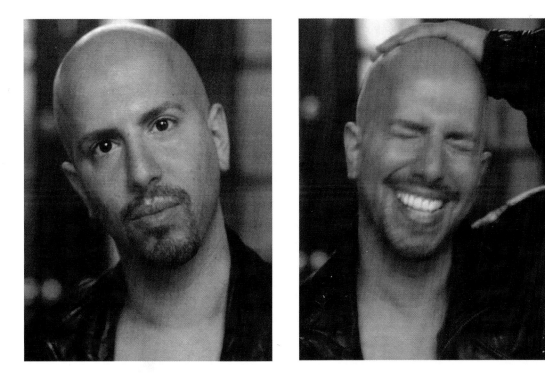

These photos are me halfway through five months of chemotherapy. Trust me, without my makeup tricks I looked like Uncle Fester from the *Addams Family*.

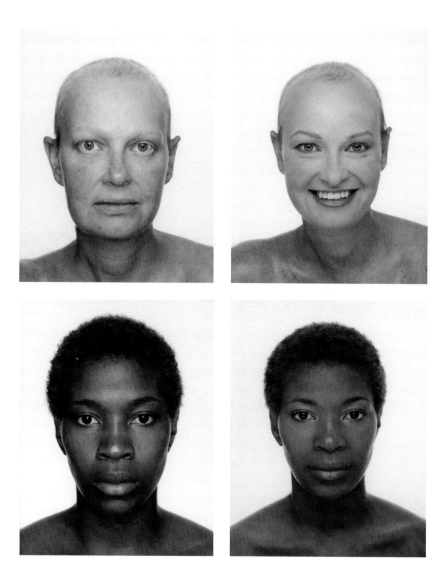

TRACEY PLEVA HILL (top) modeling the classic day face. KHADIJAH CARTER (bottom) is our minimalist, modeling the thirty-second face. She is transformed by only a foundation stick, face gloss, and mascara.

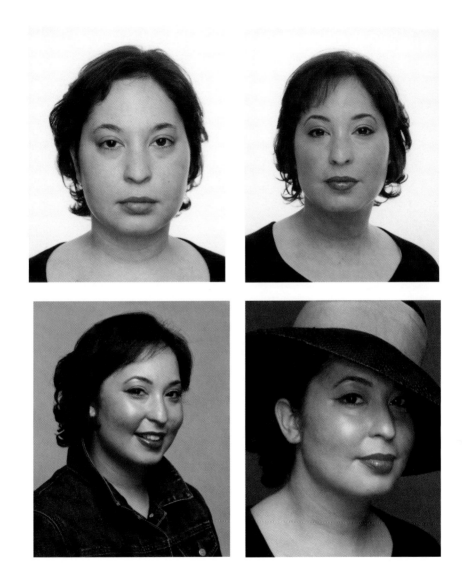

ALLISON OLSHEWITZ models my two-minute makeup (top) and how to contour your face to slim your appearance and create cheek bones (bottom). I simply added bronzer, more blush to her cheeks, and a cream shimmer high up on her cheekbones to emphasize her bone structure.

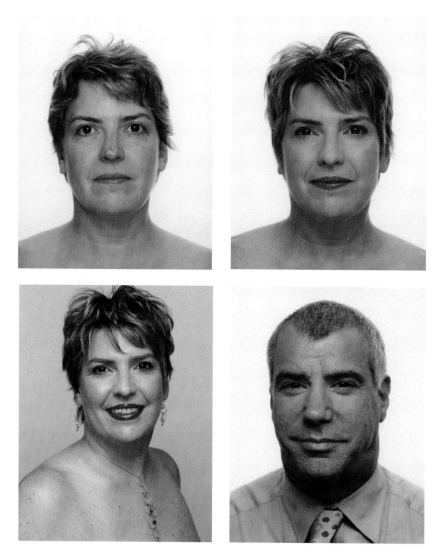

KATHY URBINA models the two-minute makeup (top) and how to take that look into evening quickly and easily (the classic evening face, bottom). I enhanced the eyeliner on her upper lash line, added a lighter-colored line to her lower lash line, then applied a rich burgundy lip gloss and added a shimmery eye gloss to her lids to take the day look into evening. JEFF BERMAN is wearing bronzer and concealer around the eyes to give his complexion a healthy glow and conceal dark circles. A great example of masculine grooming.

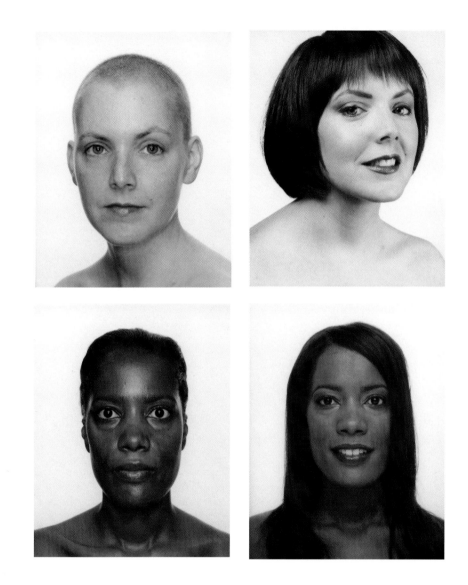

SUZANNE MURPHY (top) is wearing her own wig and the two-minute makeup.
DIANE HUGHES (bottom) is wearing the five-minute makeup.

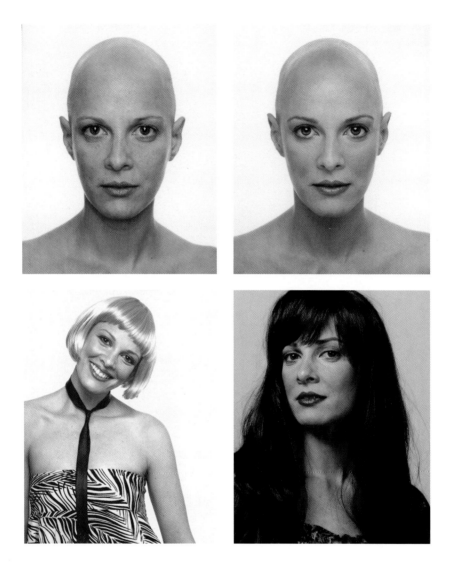

SHARON BLYNN is modeling a hybrid of the two-minute and five-minute makeup (top). I applied the two-minute makeup, then filled in her eyebrows and added eyeliner to her lower lash line. The key is to find the routine that works for you. Sharon illustrates how changing wigs and makeup can create a completely different persona (bottom).

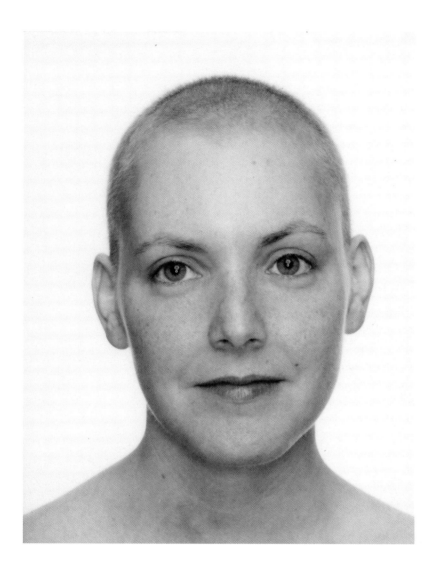

SUZANNE MURPHY as the bald bombshell. Here she is in the middle of chemotherapy about three minutes before being transformed into Marilyn Monroe. She has no makeup on, but she still looks beautiful.

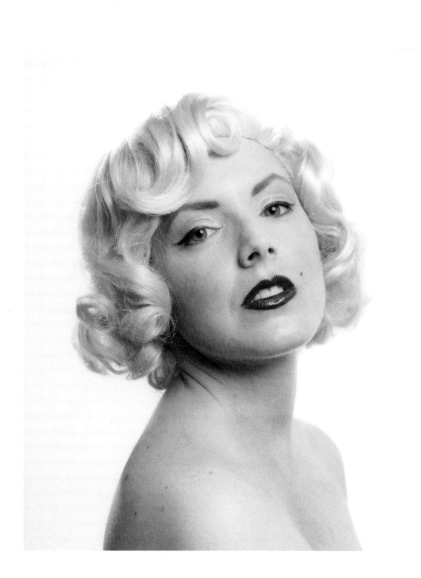

SUZANNE MURPHY as the Blonde Bombshell. I wanted to show the transformative power of makeup. Suzanne was right at the halfway point of her chemotherapy when this photo was taken. The previous picture is the beautiful Suzanne with a totally bare face.

# Six

# Covering Up Chemotherapy and Radiation Side Effects

No matter what your age or gender, there is a makeup solution that will make you look and feel better throughout the ordeal of chemotherapy. Keep in mind that when you look good, you feel better about yourself. I assure you that looking good will also help you feel better physically and help motivate you to stay connected with friends, family and coworkers. Looking your best helps not only you but also those around you to feel more at ease. The solutions here will help you put your best foot

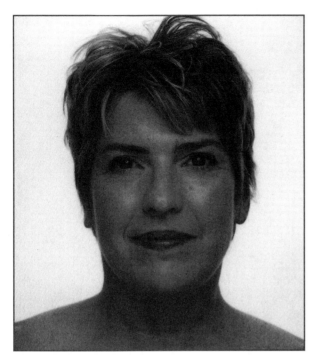

Kathy Urbina modeling the Two Minute Makeup routine. Adding bronzer and a pink blush can liven up any complexion.

forward when you're going out to dinner, going to work, seeing friends, and sharing conversation and laughs—and that can be the best medicine of all.

This chapter has specific makeup solutions for the various side effects you might experience during treatment. You may confront one or more of these side effects depending on the length and type of chemotherapy you undergo. It's important to remember that once your treatment is over, your eyelashes, hair, and eyebrows will grow back. Believe me—I had my moments during treatment when I felt like a hairless, bloated mess who would never have another romantic interest. When I look back now, I realize I did not look as bad as I thought.

## MAKEUP FOR A PALE, SALLOW COMPLEXION

1. After following the skin care regimen for your skin type (see Chapter 2 on skin care), proceed to the next step.

2. Apply bronzer in powder or liquid form. Begin with the apples of your cheeks, blending upward into the hairline (outside of eye area; see photo). Then apply bronzer to your forehead, along the hair line, along the bridge of nose, and on the chin. You want to add color wherever the sun would naturally tan you.

3. To add more dimension and color, add a flattering blush high on the cheekbone, along the hairline and over the eyes. Since you are already wearing a bronzer, avoid blush colors that are too tawny. Instead, choose a color that will give you an added glow such as soft pink, light apricot, or pale rose. The best choice to counteract the sallowness in your skin is a pink or rose blush.

4. Add a cream or powder highlighter. Apply highlighter with a subtle hand to the eyelids and outside of the eye area to top of the cheekbones. You can also apply highlighter above and below the lips. Your skin will look luminous and alive.

## CAMOUFLAGING FACIAL SWELLING AND PUFFINESS FROM STEROID USE

*When having a bad day, taking a shower and shampoo and slathering my body lotion all over really turns it around. And if I can fit it in, a little shoe shopping.*

Susan Lucci, actress

One of the side effects of steroids such as prednisone is facial swelling. The effect is cumulative, meaning that how puffy your face gets depends on your dosage and the length of time that you are required to take these medications.

While applying a bronzer can have a slimming effect on the face, you can further define, accentuate, and slim your appearance using contouring. It is one of the oldest practices in the makeup industry. These techniques have evolved over the years and now offer people even more innovative ways to use makeup to enhance the positive and eliminate or at least downplay the negative. Here are some of my suggestions for contouring the different features that I am asked about most often.

• NOSE Apply a foundation one shade darker than your skin tone (or a bronzer) on each side of your nose, carefully blending it. Then add a subtle highlighter down the center of your nose and blend.

• CHEEKBONES To enhance their cheekbones, women were traditionally told to suck in their cheeks and apply a dark color to the hollows, then a highlighter to the top of the cheekbones. Although this technique can work, it is tricky to apply and can look artificial if not expertly done. The more natural way to contour your cheeks is to smile and apply a soft, flattering color of blush from the apples of your cheeks up to your hairline. You can then apply a shimmery, neutral highlighter to the top of your cheekbones and blend.

• FACE To further slim your face, you can apply a neutral blush or powder bronzer along your entire jawline, from one ear down to your chin and up to the other ear, then blend downward toward your neck. You can apply a bit more directly under your chin. This is a photographer's trick, and it never ceases to amaze me how slimming the effect is. If you are using a liquid or gel bronzer to contour this area, simply blend a second coat of the bronzer from the jawline down over your neck.

• EYES To make your eyelids appear bigger, simply apply a medium brown eye shadow in the center of the crease of the eyelid and blend outward. Then apply a highlighter to the center of the eyelid and blend. The key to contouring is to blend, blend, blend. Although modern techniques are more subtle, it is still very important to take a moment to blend for a natural look. Once you experiment with the effects that light and dark colors can achieve, you'll find the most flattering look for your particular features.

Puffy eyes have many causes: lack of sleep, too much alcohol, salt, caffeine, and genetics. All of these can be exacerbated by stress and chemotherapy. A common issue is that as the face gets more swollen, the eyes appear to get smaller or more slanted-looking Fortunately, many remedies are available. To avoid puffiness in the first place, take preemptive measures. Avoid alcohol and salt, get a good night's sleep, and do not apply a cream moisturizer around your eyes. Instead, use a gel formula eye moisturizer (keep refrigerated for an added firming effect), which will help firm and tighten the area and reduce swelling.

If your eyes still look puffy, try any combination of the following: Rest for a few minutes with slices of cold, raw cucumber or raw potato on your eyes. Do any form of cardiovascular exercise to get your blood pumping and to help flush your system of any water you may be retaining. If all else fails, fill the sink with ice cubes and cold water, then dunk your face for thirty seconds or as long as you can stand it. Personally, I would rather live with puffy eyes than do that, but it really works.

Use makeup to conceal the puffiness and draw attention away from the problem area. Apply concealer all around your eye area (lash line to brow bone, too) and set it with powder. Then apply a dark liner and mascara to the upper lash line. This draws attention away from under-eye bags and lifts the eye. Apply a light-colored pencil such as white or pale flesh tone to the inner rim of your lower lash line. This extends the whites of your eyes, so it makes your eyes look bigger and more rounded. After applying blush, take the blush brush and sweep it over your lower eye area (yes, over the bags). This will markedly reduce their appearance.

- LIPS Whether your lips are affected by treatment or not, there are makeup tricks to help you make the most of them. To slim full or swollen lips, apply a deep shade of nonshimmery, nonglossy lipstick to the entire lip. Follow with a lip pencil that is one or two shades darker than the lipstick and line your lips, with an emphasis on lining inside your lip line to give the illusion of less full lips.

To plump up thinner lips, apply a lighter lipstick with shimmer or a glossy finish, or both. Lighter lip colors will make the lips look fuller; darker colors will make them look less full. Follow the lipstick with a lip pencil that is the exact same color as the lipstick or only one shade darker. Line the lips by lining on the lip line with an eye toward building up the lip shape to make it appear fuller. The more subtly you do this, the more realistic your fuller lip will look. Then apply a shimmery gloss to the center of your lower lip and highlighter between the peaks of your upper lip and below the center of your lower lip. This will make your lips look more full and pouty.

To tone down lips that become too pigmented during treatments, you can skip the lipstick altogether and simply apply lip balm or a clear gloss for a beautiful, finished look. If the lip pigment still appears too dark, apply a sheer nude or beige lipstick and follow with a nude pencil. Opt for a creamy, sheer, or satin finish lipstick, since your lips will probably be on the dry side. Avoid lipsticks with a matte finish. You should also avoid using lip-plumping products, since these may irritate your lips or draw more blood to the lip area, further darkening your lip color.

To amp up lip pigment that fades during treatment, which is often a symptom of dehydration and/or a lack of certain vitamins and minerals, remember that your body is fighting to rebuild itself, so you must be sure to have a well-balanced diet as much as possible and to drink plenty of water. There are also some makeup tricks you can use to alleviate pale, dry lips.

1. Exfoliate lips either by using a lip pumice or brushing lips with your toothbrush as you brush your teeth.

2. Follow with a lip balm and apply as often as possible, especially at night before going to sleep.

3. Select a lip color that is not too bright. When your lips become pale or washed out, you will find that color shows up much more strongly. So the lipstick you previously loved may not look the same during this period. Instead, choose a sheer lip color or a translucent gloss in a warm tone.

## WORKING WITH A TWO-TONE COMPLEXION CAUSED BY RADIATION TREATMENTS

In trying to even out a complexion, don't make the mistake of taking the path of least resistance by simply covering up the lighter areas of the skin to match the darker shade. On the bright side, the darker skin areas will fade in time, so your options are to either live with this problem temporarily or match the lighter tone in your complexion with a foundation that offers good coverage. But if the darker skin covers more of your face, which is common, quite a bit of effort will be required to cover the darker skin tone with a lighter shade of foundation. Thus, you may only want to go through this on special occasions if at all. My recommendation is to speak to a dermatologist to get an idea of how long it will take for your skin color to even out and to explore medicinal solutions. I had good results using 100 percent pure aloe vera gel to help radiation burns heal.

# JUST FOR TEENS

Cancer is difficult to deal with at any age, but to be diagnosed during your teen years is especially hard because life is tough enough at this time without having to deal with cancer treatments and their side effects.

The reality is, however, that people of any age can be diagnosed with cancer, and there are options for coping with the physical side effects of treatment for younger people as well. Of course, you can read all of the makeup information, selecting what you are most comfortable with as your grooming routine. But I find that the thirty-second or two-minute routines are all teenagers need, if that.

The plus side of going through treatment at such a young age is that you are physically strong, and (believe it or not) you probably look a lot prettier than you realize, since you don't have to deal with the signs of aging. What you do often have to contend with, depending on your age when diagnosed, is that your body is going through physical changes, which is something you'd have to deal with anyway. The difference is that you need to add the physical manifestations of cancer treatments into the equation, and that is a lot to handle at any age.

The thirty-second face routine is great for daytime, and upgrading to the two-minute face routine is sufficient for looking and feeling your best for special occasions. That said, I think there are essentially two things that can really make you look and feel healthy while undergoing treatment: concealer and either bronzer or tinted moisturizer (for a detailed description of these products, see Chapter 3). Here's how to use them to look your best.

## Concealer and Tinted Moisturizer

Concealer makes your eyes look less tired and hides dark circles when applied all around your eye area, from the half moon under the eyes and from the lash line up to the brow bone. If you are unsure that con-cealer will make a difference in your appearance, try applying it to just one of your eyes, then look in the mirror and marvel at the difference between your two eyes. A bronzer or tinted moisturizer will warm up your skin tone and give you a healthy flush of color.

I find that just using these two simple products can make you look and feel like you did before you began treatment. Also, keep a highlighter stick with you and apply it to eyelids, high up on the cheekbones, and to any other area for looking alive and luminous in a pinch.

## Oily Skin

Younger skin tends to be oily or acne prone. Makeup for oily or blemished skin has its own unique set of problems. Foundation and blush seem to magically turn darker about a half hour after application, and covering blemishes often seems to only draw more attention to them. But here are some general tips for an acne-prone complexion.

- Keep hair off your face. The oil and product residue from your hair products can cause skin to break out.

- Wash your hands throughout the day and avoid touching your face. Touching your face often passes dirt and bacteria onto your skin, causing breakouts.

- Keep acne cleansing pads or premoistened facial cleansing cloths on hand and clean your face immediately after coming in from outside or whenever you feel your skin getting too oily. I like Biore Cleansing Cloths or Clearasil or Oxy Acne Pads.

## Blemishes

If you are taking medication to clear your complexion, check with your oncologist to make sure it is still advisable while undergoing cancer treatments. If you are taking acne medication, your skin may be excessively dry, so choose a gel-based moisturizer to keep skin smooth. Each of the steps below will help to diminish the appearance of a blemish. Use all the tips if you have an event where your skin must look perfect or you want to wage all-out war on a pimple. When I work on a model or an actress for a photo shoot and she has a blemish that needs to be concealed, I use these surefire tricks that you can use at home to cover up that pesky pimple.

- Dab a little Visine directly on the blemish. This helps to get the red out, at least temporarily.

- If there is time, apply an astringent, witch hazel, or even rubbing alcohol directly on the blemish to dry it up as much as possible.

- Dab a drop of clay mask directly on the pimple and let it dry for five to ten minutes. A great over-the-counter mask is Queen Helene Mint Julep Mask.

- Apply an oil-free, acne-fighting moisturizer (RAMY Ultimate Therapy Cream or Clinique Oil-Free Moisturizer) after your skin is cleansed and prepped for makeup. (Even oily skin needs a moisturizer for a smoother makeup application.) If your skin is very oily, you can skip the moisturizer altogether and just use a silicone-based primer to smooth the complexion and prepare it for a makeup application.

## Makeup Especially for Oily Skin

As I said earlier, foundation darkens as it dries on oily skin. Once the oils in your skin begin to emerge, the makeup becomes wet, so the color deepens. Here are some ways to cover blemishes on oily skin.

- Try a foundation that is one shade lighter than the color you have been using.

- Keep a translucent powder compact on hand to touch up, if the problem is not terribly drastic.

- Avoid covering your face entirely with foundation, because in order to get the blemishes covered, you'll end up with an exceedingly heavy application. Instead, use a concealer or foundation stick and apply it directly on pimples and imperfections. Blend carefully with your fingers or a latex sponge and set with powder. When you are ready to add color, keep blush very light, almost nude. As it darkens (and it will), it will look perfect.

• Use eye shadows and blushes with a matte finish. Shimmer is fine for enhancing your eyes or lips only, but it only draws attention to your skin's imperfections if used on your cheeks.

## FOR MATURE SKIN

When you are more mature (or sophisticated, as we say in the beauty industry), less is more. Applying too much makeup can make you appear older by drawing more attention to fine lines and wrinkles.

The key to applying makeup when you are over fifty is to apply it strategically. The correct makeup—the most flattering colors applied in the most flattering way—can take years off of your face. The good news is that the optimum way to do this makeup routine is also the optimum way to look your best while in treatment.

It has often been said that you can tell a woman's age by the way she wears her makeup. I find this to be very true, with the exception of purchasing new colors once in a while, because most women find a routine that they like and tend to apply the makeup in the same way that they did when they first started to wear it.

When I was studying makeup in Australia, there was a very pretty thirty-something woman in my class. I asked if she, too, was looking to become a professional makeup artist. She said no, that she was perfectly happy with her career in the travel industry, but she enjoyed taking makeup classes every couple of years in order to revamp her look and see what was new and exciting in the beauty industry. I told her that she would probably be beautiful her entire life because she had such an open mind and a fresh, modern approach to her makeup routine.

### Flawless Makeup Application

Think of this as an opportunity to revamp, refine, and turbo charge your look.

• MOISTURIZE Nothing looks more aging than dry skin. Moisturized skin is softer and smoother-looking. Even the most basic moisturizer will temporarily plump up fine lines and give your complexion a more youthful appearance. Be certain to moisturize around your eyes, too. Eye moisturizers tend to be more intensive than facial moisturizers. The eyes are usually the first part of your face to show signs of age, because the skin around the eye area is the thinnest on the body and we have no oil glands in the skin just under our eyes.

- APPLY MASCARA TO THE UPPER LASH LINE ONLY This will lift your eyes. Applying mascara to your lower lash line will only drag down your eyes and draw attention to fine lines, wrinkles, or dark circles.

- APPLY EYELINER TO THE UPPER LASH LINE ONLY Nothing elicits a wow from my clients as much as when I apply eyeliner to one of their eyes and they look in the mirror and see how much more lifted, larger, and defined the lined eye looks compared to the unlined eye. Applying eyeliner is easy once you sit down and practice by applying and removing it two or three times. Practice makes perfect. (For details on applying eyeliner, read Chapter 3).

- USE A BRIGHTER LIPSTICK Brown-based colors make you look faded and dull. A bright shade will wake up your entire face.

- AVOID SHIMMERY, PEARLIZED, OR FROSTY PRODUCTS These formulas will get into the texture of your skin and emphasize lines and wrinkles. Stick to soft, matte, powdery eye shadows and blushes. If you love shimmer, then choose a shimmery lipstick or lip gloss only. Eye shadows and blush should be matte for the softest effect.

- FILL IN BROW AND LIP LINES The two features that seem to disappear with age are the eyebrow line and the lip line. You can take years off your appearance simply by filling in your eyebrows and enhancing your lip line with a lip pencil.

*Getting a pedicure at my favorite nail salon always puts me in a better mood. You are forced to stop and relax, because there's no way to get a pedicure on the go. Plus, you feel so pulled together when you have pretty toes and feet.*

Kerry Diamond, beauty director, *Harper's Bazaar* magazine

## MEN AND MAKEUP

We'll never see men clamoring around a department store makeup counter for the latest color collection. But the tide seems to be turning a bit with makeover reality television shows and the identification of metrosexuals in our society—that is, urbane and sophisticated straight men who enjoy facials, eyebrow shapings, and manicures, and love great clothes. Although we have witnessed the launch of several men's makeup lines, it still seems that makeup for men is acceptable only for actors or rock stars. That said, I must tell you that for every bride I have made up on her wedding day, I have had nearly as many grooms quietly approaching me to ask if I have makeup to cover a blemish, a scar, or that morning's razor burn—or a bronzer to give a pale complexion a much needed boost. So it's not surprising that today's men are concerned about the effects of cancer treatment on their appearance. These men face many of the same physical side effects as women. No one relishes the thought of losing eyebrows or eyelashes, or having a pasty complexion. The motivation may be different for men who are not necessarily as concerned with looking more handsome as they are with looking strong. But the empowerment from addressing these issues is the same. No one wants to look sick.

## Bronzers for Men

If I were to suggest just one product for a guy to apply during treatment, it would be bronzer. Bronzer gives the face a healthy coloring by deepening your complexion. Bronzer makes your dark circles less noticeable, even if you skip using concealer around the eyes. I recommend a liquid gel bronzer because it can be applied like a moisturizer. Start by using the lightest shade, or ask professionals at a salon or a store for their opinion on which color you should use. To be sure you use the best color, try it on first or ask for a sample.

Checking out bronzers in department stores is your best bet for samples and experienced advice. Remember, if you use a light shade, you can always apply more to intensify the color, but stay within your comfort zone. If you are not so sure about wearing makeup, apply just a little bit. Apply a drop to your forehead, each cheek, your nose, and chin. Blend it in with your fingertips. Add a drop to your neck, just below your jaw line, and blend it down and out. If well blended, no one will know you have it on. You will just look like you have a healthy complexion. For men who cringe at the thought of going to a store's cosmetic department, bronzers can also be purchased in drug stores, apothecaries, online, or even in some health food stores.

If you are pleased with the results and want to try a few more things to subtly enhance your appearance, check out the two-minute face routine, in Chapter 4.

# Seven

## Beauty Therapy Rituals

Beauty rituals—we all have them. Everything from brushing your teeth to applying makeup to stretching can be considered a beauty ritual. These rituals are important because they improve our appearance, our spirit, and our overall sense of well-being. Essentially, anything that makes you look and feel better on a regular basis can be considered a beauty ritual. You probably have some beauty rituals of your own that you're not even aware of. This chapter discusses some classic therapies and their affordable at-home alternatives to help rejuvenate, refresh, and renew you inside and out.

Although the treatments listed in this chapter are intended to improve your well-being, always check with your doctor before undertaking a body treatment. We are all different and will have different reactions to cancer treatments.

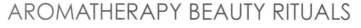

## AROMATHERAPY BEAUTY RITUALS

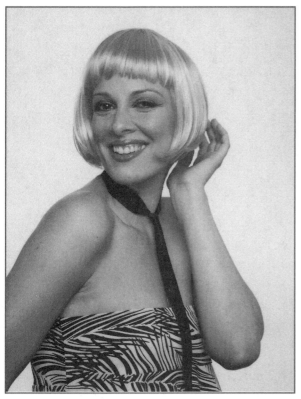

Aromatherapy can improve your mood, affect your appetite, relax you, or energize you depending on the scent. It includes everything from wearing a favorite fragrance to lighting candles, and it can become a welcome addition to your life easily and affordably. One of the stranger side effects of chemotherapy that I experienced was that my sense of smell became very sensitive to particular odors. However, I still was able to appreciate and enjoy aromatherapy. It can be a great source of comfort and pleasure during your treatment.

### Baths

*Beauty Rituals are anything that can make you feel better, relax you, and make you feel sexy.*

To unwind, swish ten to fifteen drops of the essential oil of your choice to your bath water. Immerse yourself in an exquisite experience that can be relaxing or invigorating, depending on the scent of the oil you choose. A great idea is to experiment and try mixing two or more different scents together in your bath to customize the scent and intensify the experience.

You can turn your shower and bath time into a spa experience without breaking the bank. Instead of an expensive fragranced bath oil, pour sesame, corn, almond, or even castor oil into your bath water and try a scented liquid cleanser instead of your regular soap bar. Whether or not you are on a budget, I highly recommend Dr. Bronner's 18-in-1 Pure Castile Soaps (a 32-ounce bottle costs about $5). They're available in exquisite fragrances like almond, peppermint, and eucalyptus. This multipurpose, all-natural product is truly a spa in a bottle. You can also use a homemade or commercially prepared salt or sugar body scrub to exfoliate your whole body and leave your skin smooth and silky.

## Scented Soap

Add about twenty drops total of essential oil to 4 ounces of liquid soap. Shake well before you soap up and create a lovely lather. Choose soothing scents as opposed to invigorating oils, which may be too harsh on sensitive skin. Some great-smelling natural soaps containing essential oils are available at natural food markets, or if you're up to it, make your own scented soap.

## Massage Oil or Lotion

Your skin needs additional nourishment and a soothing touch—either your own or your significant other's. Add about fifteen drops of essential oil (oil derived from plant extracts) to 1 ounce of a carrier oil (baby oil, body oil) or lotion. Apply to your entire body, focusing on any dry areas after your shower or bath. Treat yourself to a therapeutic massage and bring your own blend of massage oil or lotion with you for the massage therapist to use. This combines massage and aromatherapy and assures you that you will get to enjoy a scent you like during your session.

## Scents

Wear your favorite essential oil or add it to your favorite fragrance. Blend together. Dab on your tender spots—bend of the elbow, back of the knee, inner thigh, or anywhere you usually apply your favorite scent. If there is an essential oil you particularly like, you can layer it on to make the scent last longer. For example, if you love the scent of lavender, add some lavender oil to your favorite body wash as well as to your body lotion and fragrance. By applying the scent and layering it on while bathing, moisturizing, and then as a fragrance,

*Take time out for yourself when everything else seems to be conspiring against you, and you will start to realize that there are a lot of other positive things going on in the world.*

Valerie Latona, beauty director, *Shape* magazine

the scent will last much longer than if you apply it to only one of these options.

## Facial Mist

Add about fifteen drops of essential oil to a 2-ounce misting bottle filled with spring water. Shake and mist throughout the day. Depending on which scent of essential oil you add to the water, it can either relax or invigorate your state of mind.

## Facial Scrub

If you use a scrub, add about twelve drops of essential oil to your product, mix well, and exfoliate. Mixing in a soothing oil such as chamomile can soothe your skin as the scrub exfoliates. You can also apply just two or three drops of oil to your palm and add the scrub. This is a good way to experiment and see if you like the combination before committing to adding the scent to the entire bottle.

## Body Scrub

These scrub treatments work to eliminate toxins from the body while smoothing the skin and sloughing off dead skin using sugar or salt. Aromatic oils can be added as well to enrich the experience. Add three drops to your loofah, washcloth, or body sponge and scrub as usual. This way you will enjoy the benefits of aromatherapy as you stimulate your circulation.

There are many body scrubs to choose from: those with salt or sugar granules, cream-based, or oil based. Treat yourself to a gift basket of assorted bath and beauty products, set aside some alone time at home, then play and luxuriate. You can buy a body scrub or make your own at home by mixing baby or sesame oil with Epsom salts or sugar and your favorite aromatherapy oils.

1. Shower or bathe to clean and soften your skin.

2. Apply scrub all over your body or just on rough patches such as

your elbows and the soles of your feet. Work the scrub into your skin using gentle, circular motions.

3. Rinse the scrub off with warm water.

4. Optional: Follow with your favorite body lotion or moisturizer. Depending on the scrub you use, you may be left with a moisturizing finish from the scrub's oils that will deem moisturizer unnecessary.

## Facial Oil or Cream

Pamper your skin by enhancing your favorite oil or cream with essential oils. Add about eight drops to 1 ounce of oil or cream, mix well, and apply as usual. Again, try mixing a dollop of cream or moisturizer in your hand first with two or three drops of oil to test this out.

## Compresses

Place five drops of essential oil into a bowl of warm or cool water and mix well. Soak a washcloth and wring it out. This compress is very comforting when applied to the eye area. Use scented warm water compresses when you have a headache or want to relax. Use scented cold water compresses to reduce puffiness and bags around the eyes. Whether using a warm or cold compress, lie down for ten or fifteen minutes. When you get up, you'll feel brand new.

## Shampoo/Conditioner

Stimulate your scalp and strengthen your hair follicles. Simply add about twelve drops of essential oil to 1 ounce of mild shampoo. You can also condition your hair by adding twelve drops of essential oil to 1 ounce of conditioner, apply to your scalp and hair, and wrap with a warm towel. For healthier locks, put three drops of essential oil onto your palm and rub over the bristles of your hairbrush. Brush your hair and experience a change of mind and spirit.

## Home and Environment Fragrance

Create a mood or change the energy at home, at work, or when traveling. Use your favorite essential oils or essential oil blends in a variety of ways. Electric, candle, or clay room diffusers all work to surround you with your favorite fragrance. You can also purchase a room mist or create your own by adding fifteen to twenty drops of essential oils to a 2-ounce misting bottle filled with spring water. Shake and mist. I often use perfume, aftershave, or body sprays as room fresheners. The product doesn't have to be labeled specifically as an air freshener in order for it to work as one.

Candles are by far the best way to enjoy the benefits of aromatherapy. When I was undergoing treatment, my best friend, Michelle, sent me a box of mini-candles in assorted scents that truly improved my quality of life. I loved discovering how different scents affected my mood and sense of well-being.

# OTHER FAVORITE BEAUTY RITUALS

There are many things you can do to look and feel your best on a daily basis. They can affect you physically and mentally. Anything you do that improves your state of being can be considered a beauty ritual. Here are a few favorites.

## Exercise Therapy

Just as aromatherapy exercises your senses, working out exercises and stimulates your physical self. Which exercise you do depends on your physical state at the moment. A generation ago, cancer patients were basically encouraged not to exercise because of the misconception that if you have cancer, strenuous physical activity could wear you out. Today we know the reverse is true for most cancer patients. Of course, you should speak to your oncologist before beginning any exercise regimen.

Exercise can be very beneficial to you during treatment. Not only can exercise reduce stress and strengthen the body to ensure better recovery capabilities, but it can improve your appearance. Better circulation means a better complexion, brighter eyes and an overall look of well-being. I always think of the expression, "Use it or lose it," when I think of exercise. I think this is particularly true if you are battling to regain your health and make the most of your appearance. So speak to your doctor and then to a fitness expert. Look into establishing or maintaining the best physical fitness routine you can handle.

Many factors come into play when deciding which form of exercise is best for you. Whatever form you choose, I promise it will improve your mental and emotional well-being as well as your physical condition, because exercise leads to good health, and good health is the foundation of beauty.

*I head for the gym and a good workout. I find I can think clearly when I'm exercising. If time permits, I go right home and put on a Diana Krall CD and soak in a warm bath. That usually turns me and my mood around.*

Joy Philbin, wife of Regis Philbin and sometimes co-host

## Hair and Scalp Care

One of the world's oldest beauty rituals is hair care. Conditioning, coloring, and styling your hair also means caring for your wig, other headdress, or scalp. It's amazing how even undergoing a scalp massage or having your wig styled can make you feel good in spite of not being particularly happy about having thinner or no hair during cancer therapy. So stop feeling sorry for yourself and go have a scalp massage, or splurge on having your wig styled professionally. You'll see that I'm right.

## Makeovers

While following the tips in the makeup chapters of this book will teach you everything you'd want to know about applying your own makeup, having a complimentary makeover at a cosmetics counter is a classic beauty ritual and treat that has almost become a time-honored tradition. Learning the newest techniques and latest colors can make you more confident when you apply your own makeup at home. Just buying a new lipstick color can be a pick-me-up that will help you feel better about your appearance. Even if you feel as though the makeup artist is going to show you every product the brand ever made, keep an open mind. You could walk away with a great new color or makeup trick.

## Manicures and Pedicures

These hand and foot treatments have become a favorite pick-me-up for men and women of all ages because they are inexpensive and fun. Manicures and pedicures are also some of the easiest ways to pamper yourself if you're feeling low during cancer treatments. In addition to making your hands and feet look and feel better, they get you out of the house to socialize.

Nails often become dry and brittle during chemotherapy, and a good manicurist can recommend the most effective products to improve your nails. It is very important that you tell the manicurist if you are undergoing chemotherapy, because you may be more susceptible to infections. The manicurist can take extra precautions to ensure that tools are properly and thoroughly disinfected. Skip nail wrapping and artificial nails during chemotherapy, which will only make your dry/brittle nails worse.

## Music Therapy

We all know how music can affect us. A good beat can make you want to dance, a sad song elicits emotion, and a classical or new-age piece can relax you. When I was in warrior mode during treatment—a mindset that involves mustering up as much positive energy and will as you can to battle through the illness and side effects of treatment and come through successfully on the other side—one thing that helped me tremendously was music. When you are sick or tired, your emotions come much closer to the surface. Many others have told me that during treatment they would lose their temper much more quickly or cry at the drop of a hat. I was the same. It is a stressful and emotional time. Music affects how you feel and how you feel affects your looks.

Most powerful are the songs that I call my theme songs or mantras. My absolute favorite was a song by the group Chumbawumba called "Tubthumping." The chorus is, "I get knocked down, but I get up again, you are never going to keep me down." Combined with the driving beat of the song, these words were the powerhouse mantra that always made me feel better, stronger, and more positive when I needed a boost. Even now, the song is never far from my mind when I am having a bad day. Find a song that makes you feel the same way, whatever it is. Like aromatherapy, music can change your mood, your environment, and your energy level.

*I eat. It is all about pizza margherita for me.*

Charla Lawhon, editor-in-chief, *Instyle* magazine

## Shopping Therapy

Shopping for clothes, shoes, jewelry—anything that makes you feel good. This is also known as retail therapy. Now is the time to treat yourself. (If not now, when?) It is also a diversionary tactic. People notice when you are well dressed. If they are looking at your fabulous shoes, they are less likely to notice your hairline. This is the time for you to be selfish. Do the things that make you happy. I'm not saying that you should neglect your loved ones, but I do think that it is important during this time of adversity to put yourself first and do anything and everything that can improve your state of mind and feelings of happiness.

## Psychotherapy or Counseling

While many of the beauty rituals I have discussed are fun and offer quick gratification, I can't overlook the more serious aspect of counseling. Many people in treatment feel they have no one to turn to. So many physical and emotional issues arise during the course of a person's cancer journey. You may feel some of these issues are too embarrassing to discuss with someone close to you, or you may fear upsetting a loved one.

Finding a therapist, a counselor, or even a friend who has also been through cancer can offer you a sounding board for venting, expressing, and sharing the wide range of feelings you may be experiencing. Sharing your feelings not only may lead to getting great guidance and advice, but it will also make you feel better. There are hundreds if not thousands of support groups around the country where you can meet other people who are in similar circumstances as yourself. It can be very comforting to have an outlet for your feelings and to find a place where you feel safe to talk about your roller-coaster emotions. It is also beneficial to hear what other people are going through. This can help make you feel less alone. Many medical facilities and cancer support groups offer free one-on-one counseling. This is one beauty therapy ritual you shouldn't skip.

## Facials

A facial is a superb treat on many levels for someone living with cancer. It not only cleanses and revitalizes the skin, but just taking the time out for a facial is an excellent break to relax and unwind. There is also an added bonus: your complexion looks and feels better (we all know beauty begins with good skin). The end result is that you look better, feel rested, and are energized.

### Types of Facials

There are many different types of facials ranging from deep cleansing to firming to exfoliating. You will need to research and select the spa or dermatologist offering the particular treatment you want or need.

- CLASSIC OR BASIC FACIAL A deep pore–cleansing facial where your skin is exfoliated, massaged, steamed, and moisturized.

- HYDRATING FACIAL A step up from your basic facial where extra hydrating cleansers and moisturizers are used if your skin is dry.

- ANTIAGING FACIAL Antiaging facials use antiaging ingredients such as alpha- and beta-hydroxy acids, antioxidants such as vitamin C and vitamin A, or collagan to help diminish lines and wrinkles and give skin a healthy glow.

- ACNE-CLEARING FACIAL Acne-clearing facials incorporate gentle oil-free products that contain acne-fighting ingredients such as salicylic acid, and glycolic acid to help clear away blemishes and minimize further outbreaks.

- AROMATHERAPY FACIAL Aromatherapy facials incorporate essential oils specifically suited to your complexion's particular needs.

Aromatherapy facials are deeply relaxing. The wonderful scents make it seem like a mini-vacation.

## At-Home Facials

It's very easy to reap the benefits of a facial at home. Enjoy a facial anytime the mood strikes by following these simple steps.

1. Buy a commercially packaged mask. Choose a clay-based mask for oily skin or a cream-based mask for dry skin. There is a wide variety of masks on the market: firming, moisturizing, wrinkle-reducing, acne-reducing, to name a few. Shop around for a mask that addresses your specific needs.

2. Cleanse your face using a deep-cleaning cleanser or scrub. For sensitive skin, use a gentle, mild cleanser.

3. Pat skin dry and apply the mask to your face and neck.

4. Relax while the mask sets. Take this time to be still with your thoughts. Apply raw cucumber, raw potato slices, or an eye mask or cold compress to reduce eye puffiness.

5. Rinse off the mask and follow up with a toner or astringent designed for your skin type.

6. Follow with your moisturizer or regular skin care routine.

## Ramy's Quickie Facial On the Go

When you are in a hurry or simply not inclined to follow a full facial routine, try my fast and easy alternative.

1. Clean your face with a premoistened cleansing cloth or baby wipe.

2. Add a drop or two of your favorite firming mask to your moisturizer and apply to your face and neck.

3. Go. Follow with your makeup routine if desired.

*In the summer, I love soaking my feet in a cool bath, using a scrub, and applying a thick cream. In winter, my skin is always so dry, especially my hands. I glob on cream, then stick my hands in a pair of cotton socks, then watch some trashy reality TV.*

Rebecca Sample Gerstung, freelance beauty writer

## Laughter, the Best Beauty Therapy Ritual

Laughter is the best medicine. So rent a funny movie or go to a comedy club, read a joke book, or have lunch with friends who you enjoy. Anything you can do that will put a smile on your face is the most important beauty ritual of the day. I always say the fastest beauty trick in the world that can make you look younger, thinner, and infinitely more beautiful is to smile.

Until a cure is found for cancer, mothers are going to put on a brave front for their children, children will put on a brave face for their parents, and all cancer patients will try to face the world with strength and dignity, as difficult as that may sometimes be. Beauty, therefore, can be truly therapeutic, because the new definition of beauty is not necessarily striving for physical perfection but rather making the most of who you are and feeling great about it. This is never more important than when you are confronted with cancer. Your physical and inner beauty are challenged. Beauty therapy can be your secret weapon—an asset that helps you not just survive this difficult time but thrive with grace and personal style!

# RESOURCES

These organizations are dedicated to helping men, women, and children who are facing cancer.

## AMERICAN CANCER SOCIETY

1-800-ACS-2345

www.cancer.org

The American Cancer Society is an international organization dedicated to the fight against cancer through research, public policy, community services, and support groups to help educate the public about cancer prevention, early detection, treatment, survival, and quality of life.

## CANCERCARE

275 Seventh Avenue

New York, NY 10001

1-800-813-HOPE

www.cancercare.org

CancerCare is a national nonprofit organization that provides free professional support services to anyone affected by cancer: people with cancer, caregivers, children, loved ones, and the bereaved. CancerCare programs—including counseling, education, financial assistance, and practical help—are provided by trained oncology social workers and are completely free of charge.

## COSE BELLE

15 Oak Street

Staten Island, NY 10305

718-482-3575

718-815-0666 (fax)

info@cosebelle-ny.com (email)

www.cosebelle-ny.com

Cose Belle is a website boutique specifically designed for women dealing with breast cancer. Cose Belle is geared toward offering a more comfortable life postsurgery and provides high-quality postmastectomy lingerie, swimwear, breast prostheses, cosmetics, and accessories for breast cancer survivors.

## G & P FOUNDATION FOR CANCER RESEARCH

41 East 11th Street, 11th Floor
New York, NY 10003
212-905-6202
www.GPFoundation.com
The G & P Foundation for Cancer Research encourages the development of more effective therapies for patients with leukemia, lymphoma, and related cancers. The foundation funds research to improve the efficacy of cancer treatments, reduce their toxicity, and improve the quality of life for patients with leukemia or lymphoma.

## SUSAN G. KOMEN BREAST CANCER FOUNDATION

5005 LBJ Freeway, Suite 250
Dallas, TX 75244
972-855-1600
National toll-free help line: 1-800-I'M AWARE (1-800-462-9273)
www.susangkomen.org
With over 75,000 volunteers and 100 affiliates, the Susan G. Komen Foundation is dedicated to eradicating breast cancer through fund-raising for research to find a cure and support community-based education, screening, and treatment programs.

## NATIONAL CHILDREN'S LEUKEMIA FOUNDATION

172 Madison Avenue
New York, NY 10016
212 686-2722
Outside New York: 1-800-GIVE-HOPE
www.leukemiafoundation.org
The NCLF is one of the largest non profit organizations in the fight against leukemia and cancer in children and adults. NCLF's main objective is to provide the cure for children and adults, and to ease the family's burden during their hospital stay. NCFL offers a wealth of information on the latest breakthroughs in treatment, a support network with other families who have gone through similar ordeals, and a "Make a dream come true" program to fulfill the wishes of any child with a life-threatening illness anywhere in the country.

## SHOP WELL WITH YOU

38 Greene Street, 4th Floor
New York, NY 10013
212-226-0466
www.shopwellwithyou.org

Shop Well with You is a not-for-profit organization that helps women with a history of cancer improve their quality of life by using clothing as a creative means toward wellness. SWY offers information and resources; outreach programs called Fashion Your Own Sense of Self, which take place in hospitals and support organizations; and one-on-one personalized assistance. By providing these confidence-building tools free of charge, SWY helps to facilitate the healing process.

## YOUNG SURVIVAL COALITION

155 6th Avenue, 10th Floor
New York, NY 10013
212-206-6610
www.youngsurvival.org

The Young Survival Coalition is the only international nonprofit network of breast cancer survivors and supporters dedicated to the concerns and issues unique to young women and breast cancer. Through action, advocacy, and awareness, the YSC seeks to educate the medical, research, breast cancer, and legislative communities and to persuade them to address breast cancer in women age forty and under. YSC also serves as a point of contact for young women living with breast cancer.

# FURTHER READING

WHY I WORE LIPSTICK TO MY MASTECTOMY by Geralyn Lucas
(St. Martin's Press)
The author, a breast cancer survivor, shares her experience in a touching yet funny book that shares the empowerment she felt in looking her best through the trials and tribulations of treatment.

BODY & SOUL: THE COURAGE AND BEAUTY
OF BREAST CANCER SURVIVORS by Jean Karotkin
(Emmis Books).
This book shares inspirational and poignant stories of cancer survivors and the incredible measures they took in various ways to survive cancer and thrive.

BREAST CANCER HUSBAND: HOW TO HELP YOUR WIFE (AND YOURSELF) DURING DIAGNOSIS, TREATMENT AND BEYOND
by Marc Silver (Rodale, Inc.)
The author shares his experience as the husband of a woman diagnosed with cancer, the emotional repercussions on a couple during diagnosis, and the best way to cope and support each other during treatment.

# THE MODELS—BEAUTY THERAPISTS

The models shown in the photos in this book are cancer survivors. When they heard I was writing a book on beauty tips for cancer survivors and was looking for models, they enthusiastically volunteered their time and energy to help with this project. Their willingness to lend support to this project is indicative of the fact that they are each inspirational in their own way. They are all now counted among my friends, and I probably never would have met any of them had our lives not been touched by cancer.

JEFFREY BERMAN I met Jeff at a Race for the Cure charity event a few months after I finished treatment. We were introduced as fellow cancer warriors and became instant friends. I told him I had just finished treatment and asked when he had. He replied, "I never finish." The thought never occurred to me that someone might have a chronic battle to fight, as my own experience was punctuated by having a very definite beginning, middle, and end.

Jeff was very physically fit when he was diagnosed with chronic lymphocytic leukemia in 1990, and he found that participating in everyday activities and exercise helped him in his fight against cancer. He ran marathons before he was diagnosed and saw no reason to stop afterward. (I always tell Jeff that I did not run marathons before I had cancer, I did not run during treatment, and the only way he will get me to run now is if he chases me with a gun.) In 1994, Berman and Fred Lebow, founder of the New York Road Runners Club, established the first exercise support group for people with cancer, which became the FORCE (Focus on Rehabilitation and Cancer Education) program a few years later. FORCE teaches cancer patients how they can help themselves by making gradual lifestyle changes in exercise, diet, and stress management. This philosophy does not claim that doing so will cure cancer, but it suggests that patients will be in a better position to fight cancer when they strengthen their bodies and minds in conjunction with cancer treatments prescribed by their doctors. Today, Jeff is happily married and has a baby on the way. People always say that champion cyclist Lance Armstrong is a hero and an inspiration. I tell Jeff that he is my Lance Armstrong.

SHARON BLYNN I met Sharon recently when I received the Inspiration Award at the Michael Awards, a benefit for the National Children's Leukemia Foundation. There were several runway shows during the evening honoring designers such as Louis Vuitton and Petit Bateau. I was watching one of the shows when a striking, gorgeous, bald model strutted down the runway with such presence that I was not sure if she was striking because she was bald or because of the confidence with which she strutted down the runway. Later, as I was returning to my table after accepting my award, Sharon came over and introduced herself. We bonded immediately, and I think only about three seconds passed before I asked her to participate in this book.

Sharon was diagnosed in 2000 with a rare form of ovarian cancer. She chose to use this experience to share with others what she learned about having a positive attitude, making healing choices, and applying self-love and self-empowerment to overcome her health crisis by founding the Bald Is Beautiful organization (www.baldisbeautiful.org).

KHADIJAH CARTER I met Khadijah at a charity event for the Young Survival Coalition the night before we shot the photographs for this book. A natural beauty with cheekbones I'd kill for, Khadijah has a seven-year-old child and is a recent breast cancer survivor. She epitomizes the modern woman who has lived with cancer and has not let it dim her spirit, her appearance, or her confidence. She is a great role model to others, which is why I had to have her model for this book.

DIANE HUGHES Diane was a client of mine for several years. One day she called to ask me some questions about treatments and support groups for cancer patients. She had been diagnosed with breast cancer.

In fact, she had been misdiagnosed for over a year before finally discovering that she had cancer. As a result of her misdiagnosis, the cancer had spread and her journey was much tougher than it needed to be. Yet every time I saw Diane, she seemed serene and at peace, always with a smile on her face and an easy laugh. She survived that cancer experience and went right back to embracing life. A few months ago, she told me she was diagnosed with a recurrence of breast cancer, but this time it was caught very early, thanks to the diligence of regular checkups.

Had she not told me, I would never have known that she was going through the whole ordeal again. She continues to be as calm, cool, and collected as ever. She made a choice to get through it gracefully and she has, which is why she elicits such admiration from me.

SUZANNE MURPHY Suzanne came to see me for a private makeup lesson on the recommendation of a mutual friend. All I knew about her was that she was a young woman undergoing treatment for breast cancer. In walked this sunny beauty with a contagious smile and an amazingly positive attitude. I honestly felt she did not need any makeup help or beauty tips from me because she already looked terrific. Suzanne felt it would give her a confidence boost and simply make her feel better to get some makeup pointers, so we had a fun session together. When she left, I felt as though my mood and mindset had gotten a lift. That is how great her energy was.

ALLISON OLSHEWITZ About two or three years ago, I arrived at CancerCare in New York to teach one of my Beauty Master Classes. I headed to the conference room where I usually teach my class. Allison (Ali) had taken off her hat and was about to try on a wig. I excused myself, feeling mortified that I might have embarrassed her, and I quickly exited the room. As it turned out, Ali was there to attend my class that day. She was only twenty-three and had recently been diagnosed with acute myelogenous leukemia. She looked like a sixteen-year-old Audrey Hepburn. After the class, I apologized for walking in on her as she was trying on wigs. She laughed and completely put me at ease because it was a nonissue for her. She just emanated positive energy and has at every encounter I have had with her.

TRACY PLEVA HILL Tracy was a client at one of my makeup classes. At the time, she was a thirty-two-year-old mother who was diagnosed with breast cancer shortly after her son's first birthday. Because of her young age, her cancer was not recognized and treated by her doctors until it had metastasized. She was undergoing treatment and was bald and had no eyebrows. But the lack of hair couldn't conceal her lovely features. Still, she was happy to see her eyebrows again, even if they were the product of a makeup application.

Tracy has since undergone surgery to remove a brain tumor and is currently undergoing chemotherapy, four years after originally being diagnosed. She works full time and is a wonderful wife and mother. Despite all her adversity, Tracy is just so cool that even through her anger she finds humor in everything. It is said that when someone is burned by adversity, she is either broiled to bitterness or burnished to gold. Tracy is pure gold.

KATHY URBINA Kathy was diagnosed with cancer in January 2004 and is in the midst of treatment after having a double mastectomy and reconstruction. Kathy is an amazing example for her daughter because of her positive attitude and the strength she exhibits during treatment. Cancer has not dimmed her passion and sense of purpose one bit: she remains dedicated to saving children in China who have been orphaned by AIDS.

# INDEX

# ABOUT THE AUTHOR

Ramy began his career in beauty after graduating magna cum laude from St. John's University, then dropping out of law school and relocating to Sydney, Australia, to attend the Sydney College of Makeup Art and the Napoleon Academy of Beauty. This career change offered Ramy the opportunity to pursue freelance work as a professional makeup artist, traveling through Singapore and Europe and back to his hometown of New York City before taking a job as a makeup artist for Bobbi Brown.

In 1997, Ramy was diagnosed with non-Hodgkin's lymphoma. Fortunately, the cancer was caught early and he triumphed with a full recovery after six months of chemotherapy and radiation treatments. Like millions of others, Ramy suffered the physical repercussions of those treatments and personally experienced the limited amount of help available to cancer patients dealing with the physical evidence of chemotherapy and radiation. Through his own experience and by speaking to people in the industry, he discovered how beneficial it would be to write a beauty guidebook that offered expert advice on how to conceal the physical side effects of cancer treatments. And so the *Beauty Therapy* book idea was born. This in turn led to the creation of the RAMY beauty therapy product line, which launched at Bergdorf Goodman in 1998 and is now sold nationwide in select department stores and boutiques.

Ramy's philosophy is simple: minimum makeup, maximum impact! If you select the correct color palette to enhance your features and apply it correctly, you can look younger and more beautiful with a minimum of products and effort. This viewpoint keeps Ramy busy, as he continues to see clients while working on the development of the RAMY beauty therapy product collection. His ability to select optimum colors for each individual as well as dramatically lift the eye with his gift for eyebrow shaping has been written up in the pages of every major fashion and beauty magazine—*Vogue, Allure, InStyle, Self,* and *Town & Country.* Ramy's work has also been seen on national television shows including the *Oprah Winfrey Show, E! Entertainment Television's Fashion File,* and *Entertainment Tonight.* Ramy's looks have also graced the runways of recognizable fashion shows such as Valentino and XOXO.

Known as the "Willy Wonka" of the beauty world, Ramy strives to bring innovative formulas and products to the market. RAMY beauty therapy incorporates Ramy's minimum makeup, maximum impact! philosophy with his holistic approach to well-being. The entire multipurpose product line is formulated with antioxidant vitamins, avocado oil, and sunscreens. The oil-free powder formulations are silicone treated and micronized for incredible wear and a lightweight feel. Most incredibly, this basic face collection is suitable for any skin tone, from the lightest to the darkest complexions. The line includes an array of the best of the basics—products and colors that can create a variety of glamorous and wearable looks for everyone.

Overall, Ramy is known for his humor, honesty, and creative mind. As long as he is helping people bring out their individual beauty and ability to feel good about themselves while creating innovative and unique products, he will continue to rock the beauty industry! Now cancer-free for seven years, Ramy lives in Manhattan with his cat, Arlo, and is the proud uncle of Maya Hanna Ron.